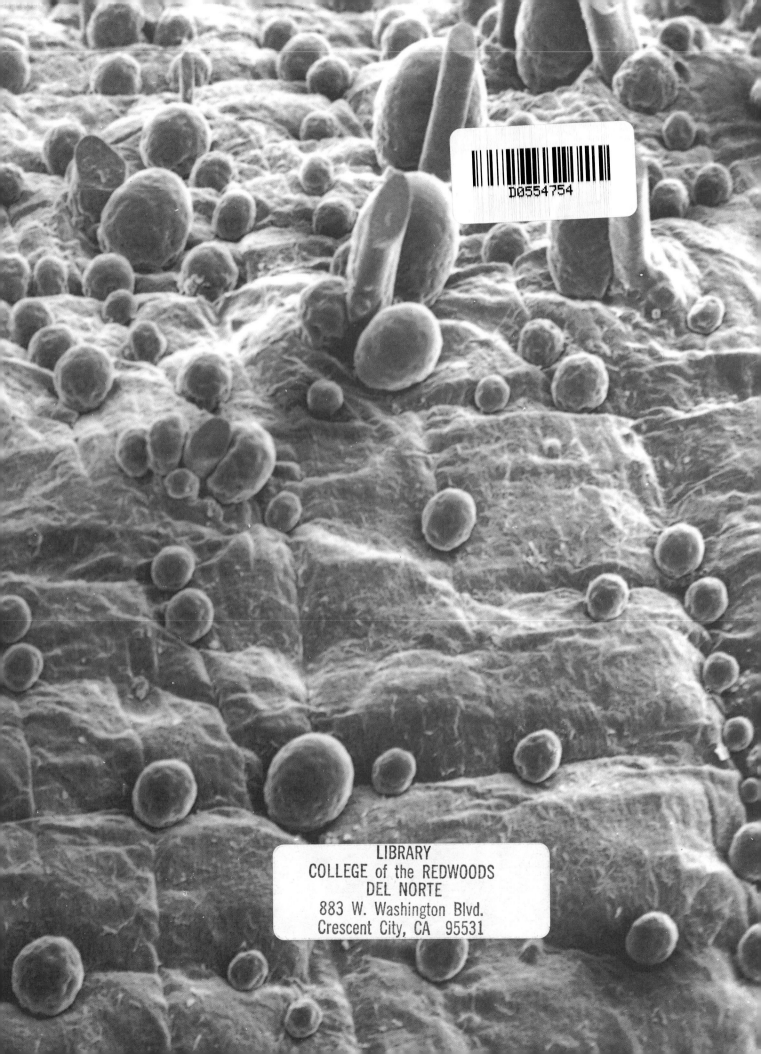

Atlas of Normal
Human Skin

Atlas of Normal Human Skin

William Montagna   Albert M. Kligman

Kay S. Carlisle

With 180 Plates in 484 parts, 308 in Full Color

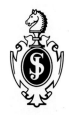

Springer-Verlag
New York Berlin Heidelberg London Paris
Tokyo Hong Kong Barcelona Budapest

William Montagna, PhD
Oregon Regional Primate
    Research Center
Beaverton, OR 97006, USA

Albert M. Kligman, MD, PhD
University of Pennsylvania
    School of Medicine
Philadelphia, PA 19104, USA

Kay S. Carlisle, MS
Oregon Regional Primate
    Research Center
Beaverton, OR 97006, USA

Histological Technician: Nicholas A. Roman, Oregon Regional Primate Research Center, Beaverton, OR 97006, USA
Medical Illustrator: Joel Ito, Oregon Regional Primate Research Center, Beaverton, OR 97006, USA

Supported by grants from the Foundation for Basic Cutaneous Research and the Ortho Pharmaceutical Corporation

Frontcover: Surface of papillary dermis (see Plate 58).
Front endsheet: Replica of the surface of the junction of the vermilion border of the lip (without hairs) and the cutaneous surface (with hairs). The round vesicles are trapped sweat bubbles. SEM.
Back endsheet: The undersurface of the epidermis of the toe of a 6-year-old child is a mirror image of the epidermal outer surface.

Library of Congress Cataloging-in-Publication Data
Montagna, William.
    Atlas of normal human skin / by William Montagna, Albert M.
Kligman, Kay S. Carlisle ; histological technician, Nicholas A.
Roman ; medical illustrator, Joel Ito.
      p. cm.
    Includes bibliographical references and index.
    ISBN 0-387-97769-4. — ISBN 3-540-97769-4
    1. Skin—Anatomy—Atlases. I. Kligman, Albert M., 1916– .
II. Carlisle, Kay S. (Kay Susan) III. Title.
    [DNLM: 1. Skin—anatomy & histology—atlases. WR 17 M758a]
QM484.M66 1992
611′.7—dc20
                                                91-5225

Printed on acid-free paper.

Production managed by Bill Imbornoni; manufacturing supervised by Rhea Talbert.
Media conversion by Bytheway Typesetting Services, Norwich, NY.
Printed and bound by Times Offset Ltd., Singapore.
Printed in Singapore.

9 8 7 6 5 4 3 2 1

ISBN 0-387-97769-4 Springer-Verlag New York Berlin Heidelberg
ISBN 3-540-97769-4 Springer-Verlag Berlin Heidelberg New York

To Leona, Lori, and Mike

PREFACE

It is the fashion today for many biological scientists to decry anatomical studies as merely "descriptive" and so archaic as to be ignored by eager molecular biologists as they push forward the frontiers of scientific knowledge. This short-sighted view betrays an ignorance of the indispensable role of morphology in the continuing growth of the biomedical sciences. When Watson and Crick reported their discovery of the double helix of DNA, they basically "described" the structure of that extraordinary molecule. The masters of biology did not suffer from this prejudice.

It behooves us to know our roots. All biologists should know Max Schultze (1825–1874), the so-called father of modern biology, and Theodor Schwann (1810–1882), for whom Schwann cells are named and who, together with M. Schleiden (1804–1881), was responsible for that master stroke of generalization, the *cell theory*, published in 1838 in the Paris Academy of Sciences. Unfortunately, the details of the cell theory were buried in Schwann's ponderous 1839 German article under the loosely translated title "Microscopical Investigations of the Structure and Growth of Animals and Plants," spread out over 215 octavo pages.

Anatomy (morphology) is the study of architecture: how living systems are organized. It covers a broad range: from the grossly visible to the submicroscopic and right down to the macromolecules that can now be visualized with specific antibodies.

The task of anatomy is to read function out of design. Szent-Györgyi once remarked, "There is no real difference between structure and function; they are two sides of the same coin. If structure does not tell us anything about function, it means we have not looked at it correctly."

Skin is an attractive organ for basic biomedical studies. In studying skin, the biochemist or the immunologist who does not appreciate its architectural complexity may fall on his or her face. Many a clever report is rendered worthless because the authors did not understand that the original skin sample contained a variety of distinct tissues that may have contaminated the results. For example, although about 50% of the weight of the epidermis is made up of dead stratum corneum, some scientists believe they are studying only living epidermal cells.

Histology has ancient origins. Its most important transition occurred in 1673 with the first publication by the Dutchman, Leeuwenhoeck (1632–1723). In that paper he casually mentioned the construction of the small, simple, two-lens microscope with which he made his observations. It is possible that Leeuwenhoeck did not foresee the great impact on biological sciences that his microscope would have. Later, the pioneering work of Bichat (1771–1801) opened up a grand era of microscopic studies. Following his treatises, many new theories were formulated during the nineteenth century in Germany, France, England, and Italy. These early theories established the foundations for the twentieth-century explosion of biological discoveries. New technologies during this century have enabled anatomists to peer ever deeper into the recesses of the cells. A tidal wave of discovery occurred during the early half of the twentieth century with the introduction of histochemistry, an assemblage of disciplines that attempted to identify the chemical composition of cells and tissues. Histochemistry was at first bewildering, leading to so many strange results that the Seattle pathologist Russel Ross called it histoalchemy. Histochemistry led to cytochemistry, which, aided by the refinements of biochemical and immunological techniques, gave rise to immunocytochemistry, which could be studied with both light and electron microscopes.

At about midcentury all eyes were opened wide by the majestic high resolution of the electron microscope. The pioneers in electron microscopy had difficulties in correctly identifying the extraordinary structures they saw. It took a number of years before these observations could be correlated with structures previously shown with the light microscope. New techniques had to be invented for the fixation of tissues and for the cutting of ultrathin sections. The race for the first publication led to a profusion of curious revelations that could not be confirmed. Some pundits prophesied that a special journal, *Acta Artifacta*, should be created for electron microscopists. It took some decades to sort out the conflicts and the confusion.

The next impressive event in the study of tissues was the development of the scanning electron microscope, which added three-dimensional perspectives and created views of inestimable beauty.

One has the feeling that perhaps the ultimate in structural details has been achieved. Moreover, today most structures that have been identified have also been characterized functionally and biochemically. Each month brings to light new details of ultrastructure. Students trained only in chemistry cannot appreciate the complexity of the organization of, for example, the basement membrane of the skin. Scientific inquiry and specialization generates ignorance as rapidly as it accumulates new knowledge.

Morphologic revelations are aired daily and the old adage has been proven. Anatomy does determine physiology. No educated biomedical student can afford to be indifferent to structure.

WILLIAM MONTAGNA
ALBERT M. KLIGMAN
KAY S. CARLISLE
March 1992

ACKNOWLEDGMENTS

So many people helped us in preparing this Atlas that it is not possible to acknowledge all of them, but we can single out some of them. The Foundation for Basic Cutaneous Research (FBCR) and Ortho Pharmaceutical Corporation supported this project. We are grateful to Mr. Les Riley for his boundless help. The Procter and Gamble Company was generous in allowing us to use materials that we had developed especially for them. Among the many people who helped us at Procter and Gamble, we salute Drs. Sergio Baranovsky, Stephen Kirchner, and Vladimir Gartstein. Nicholas Roman prepared nearly all of the histological material that we photographed. Our respective spouses, Leona, Lori, and Mike, were cheerful, patient, and understanding. We also thank Brianna and David for their willingness to share their "mom" with her work. The Oregon Regional Primate Research Center (ORPRC) and the Medical Research Foundation of Oregon (MRFO) put all of their facilities at our disposal. Drs. Frank Parker and Francis Storrs and the Dermatology Department at the University of Oregon Health Sciences Center were most cooperative in helping us obtain biopsy specimens. All of the scientists who contributed illustrations did so with cheerful words. None of these were more helpful to us than Dr. Irvin Braverman of Yale University Medical School and Dr. W. H. Fahrenbach of the ORPRC. Mr. Joel Ito, medical illustrator of the ORPRC, executed the diagrams used in the Atlas. We are grateful to Bernice Marcks for many favors, large and small.

CONTENTS

PLATES

Plates

Hair and Hair Follicles

Hypodermis

INTRODUCTION

An ancient Chinese proverb says that a picture is worth more than ten thousand words. Word pictures do not convey the specificity of actual images. Pictures, more than words, convey what one wants to demonstrate.

All of the illustrations in this Atlas, the first of its kind, are of human skin. We have avoided illustrating the skin of other mammals, not because we think that comparative anatomical studies have no value, but because the subject is too vast. We have shown "normal," nonpathological human skin from different parts of the body of men and women, children and fetuses, of various ages and different races. The illustrations in this volume indicate how skin differs in the various regions of the body. For example, although the entire body is covered with an epidermis, that tissue is very different over the axilla, the lips, the fingers, the eyelids, and the genitalia. At each site, the anatomical organization matches function with structure. We have searched in vain for a perfect epidermis, which is at best an abstraction designed for the beginner. A perfect epidermis, probably, exists only in histology textbooks. In medicine, the normal is the key to understanding the abnormal. However, the range of normalcy is wide, and all too often pathology is read into a specimen that falls within the spectrum of normal variation.

We do not cite references, because this is a picture gallery of the structure of human skin and not a literature source. And we do not describe histological techniques; there are many good texts that describe the technical procedures in scrupulous detail. The citation of the original magnification (OM) in the illustration legends tells only about a tactical point.

We have generally identified the embedding media, the thickness of the section, and the stain used. For light microscopy, the preservation of specimens that are embedded in methacrylate is generally superior to those embedded in paraffin and allows thinner sections to be cut. The thickness of histological sections is always a concern to histologists, whose general aim is to cut sections as thin as possible. Such an aim has merits, but thicker sections are often more helpful in the study of the paths of fibers, nerves, and blood vessels. The thickness of sections also influences staining. Sections on the same slide may vary in thickness due to the unavoidable variation that occurs in microtome sectioning. Consequently thicker sections stain more intensely than thinner ones. Different stains give different information about tissues and cells. Also, the staining

1

results are often pH-dependent. Hale's colloidal iron technique, for example, stains mucus well at alkaline or acidic pH values, but proteoglycans stain only at certain pH values.

The various technologies we have presented emphasize both instrumental advances and technical achievements. In addition to the light microscope, modern histological methods require the use of complicated optical instruments, which include the transmission electron microscope (TEM) and the scanning electron microscope (SEM); each has advantages as well as limitations. They complement each other and show different aspects of the same structures. Histochemistry has also advanced the findings of light microscopy considerably since midcentury. The science of histology has borrowed techniques from biochemistry and immunology. The technological developments turn up new insights at a dizzying rate that help put the puzzle of skin together; anatomy and physiology are now closer together than ever before.

There is order and beauty in living forms. Conrad Gesner (1516–1565), a Swiss physician of remarkable erudition, who translated into Latin scientific works on natural history from the Greek, Arabic, and Hebrew, all published in 20 volumes, was such a champion of fine illustrations that the four volumes of his *Historia Animalium* contain the very best woodcuts of the 16th century. For example, Albert Dürer's picture of the rhinoceros is by no means the best illustration in Gesner's work. Gesner was also a devoted physician who took care of plague victims and died himself of the plague at the age of 49. We believe Gesner might have enjoyed this book. Marcello Malpighi (1628–1694), a physician from Bologna who made many discoveries on the anatomy of skin, might also have appreciated this Atlas.

A seldom stressed point in histology is the esthetic value of things in nature. Preparations of skin can be esthetic delights. There is an orderly pattern of things in nature, and good histological preparations should reflect beauty and order.

Overview of Skin

The skin consists of an outer epidermis, the dermis, and the hypodermis. It includes nerves, blood vessels, glands, and hair follicles. The numerous components of skin are responsible for its varied functions; these include protection from the external environment, inhibition of water loss, absorption and blockage of radiation, temperature regulation, sensory perception, and immunological surveillance.

PLATE 1

DIAGRAM of SKIN ARCHITECTURE

The diagram shows all of the various structures in the skin; however, nowhere in normal skin are all these structures found together.

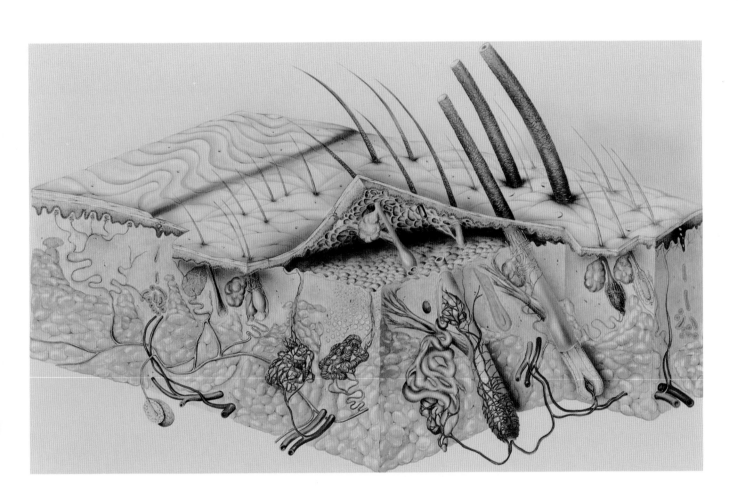

Epidermis

The epidermis, the outermost part of the skin, is a continually renewing, stratified, squamous epithelium which has remarkable biological properties. The epidermis was first described by Marcello Malpighi (1628–1694), who believed that it was a gelatinous membrane, and divided it into an inner layer of viable cells (now known as the stratum malpighii) and an outer one of anucleated horny cells (stratum corneum). Most of the cells in the epidermis are keratinocytes arranged in layers that represent different stages of their differentiation. The outer layer, the horny layer, is a layer of extraordinary properties, and functions as a barrier. It protects the body from the environment and helps maintain the internal milieu.

PLATE 2

DERMATOGLYPHICS

The plantar and palmar surfaces are filigreed by alternating ridges and sulci; the details of these configurations and markings are known collectively as dermatoglyphics. The permanence of dermatoglyphics makes them uniquely useful for personal identification. Each body area has surface markings that are specific for that region and for that individual.

Ridges range in length from "islands," containing only one pore or orifice of a sweat gland, to long extended lines that may branch and that often follow arched sweeps that form recognizable patterns. At the fingertips, the principal designs are whorls, loops, arches, and combinations of these. Whenever three ridge patterns come together from opposite directions, they form triangular patterns called triradia.

A. The dermatoglyphics in the index finger of a 32-year-old man show a mixed pattern that combines a loop and an arch. OM 5x. Courtesy of Prof. Antonio Tosti.

B. The whorl dermatoglyphics pattern in this index finger of a 78-year-old farmer is crisscrossed by grooves that on fingerprints show up as "white lines." White lines or imperfections are nearly always present in the dermatoglyphics of older people but can also be present in young people. OM 15x. Courtesy of Prof. Antonio Tosti.

C. This sharp whorl pattern is from the thumb of a 30-month-old child. Children, who have small hands and fingers, also have small dermatoglyphics. The width of the furrows increases at the same rate as the growth of the hands. The fingerprints of women are usually smaller than those of men, who have larger hands and fingers. OM 15x. Courtesy of Prof. Antonio Tosti.

D. The way the hands have been used in a lifetime has an impact on the intactness of dermatoglyphics. These dermatoglyphics are nearly wiped out in the index finger of an 86-year-old mason. Both age and use and/or abuse have brought on this abnormality. OM 15x. Courtesy of Prof. Antonio Tosti.

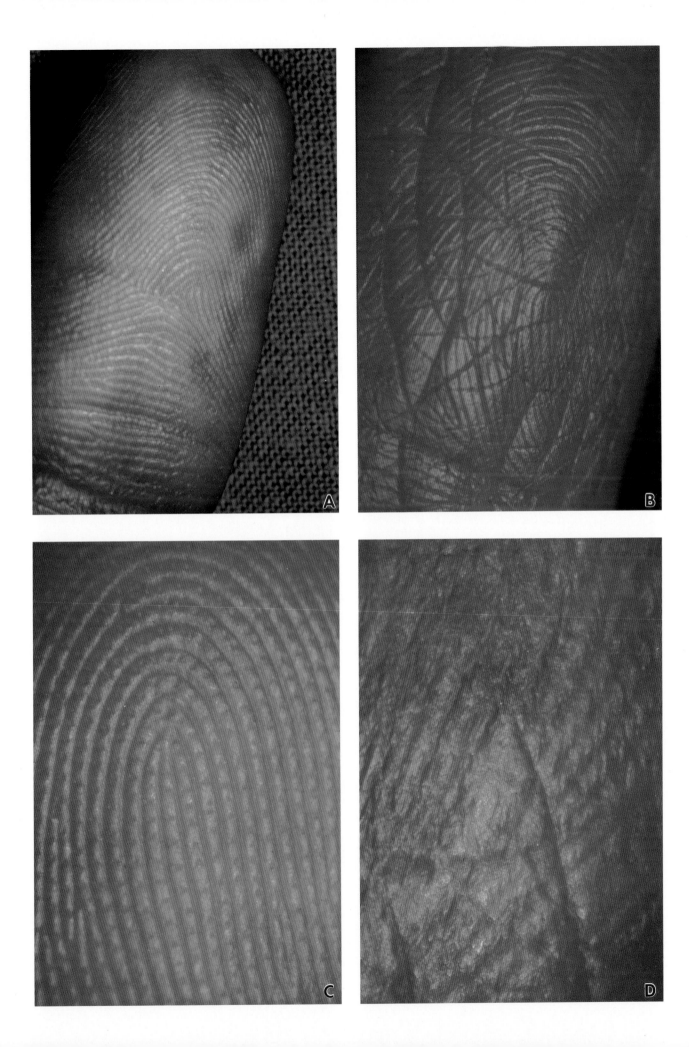

PLATE 3

SKIN MICROTOPOGRAPHY

The entire outer surface of the skin is imprinted with patterned intersecting lines similar to dermatoglyphics, which are unique to the area where they are found and are not identical in any two individuals. These figures of intact skin from the back of the hand are photographed through a skin microscope at an original magnification of 16x. They show the changes in surface microtopography that occur with maturation and aging. Courtesy of Prof. Antonio Tosti.

A. Microtopography of the back of the hand of a 16-year-old boy.

B. The microtopography is largely wiped out in this hand of a 75-year-old man. Wrinkles are evident (arrow). Hairs develop in late adolescence and become very coarse in old age.

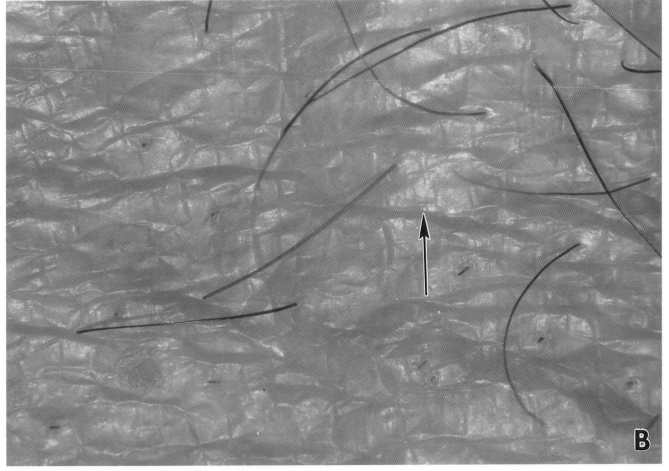

PLATE 4

SKIN SURFACE

Flexure lines, ridges, furrows, and folds are formed in characteristic patterns during fetal life. The patterns remain largely unchanged during the lifetime of the individual; they are altered somewhat with age and external insults such as sunlight.

A. SEM micrograph of a silicone replica of the surface of the forearm of an infant. The round globules may be lipid droplets. Even though an infant's skin is smooth and looks patternless to the naked eye, it has an elaborate and uniform microrelief. OM 90x. Courtesy of Prof. R. Caputo, Dr. Mauro Barbareschi, and Dr. Marcello Calvi.

B. SEM micrograph of a silicone replica of the surface of the forearm of an old man. The microrelief is mostly flattened out, irregular, and in disorder. OM 120x. Courtesy of Prof. R. Caputo, Dr. Mauro Barbareschi, and Dr. Marcello Calvi.

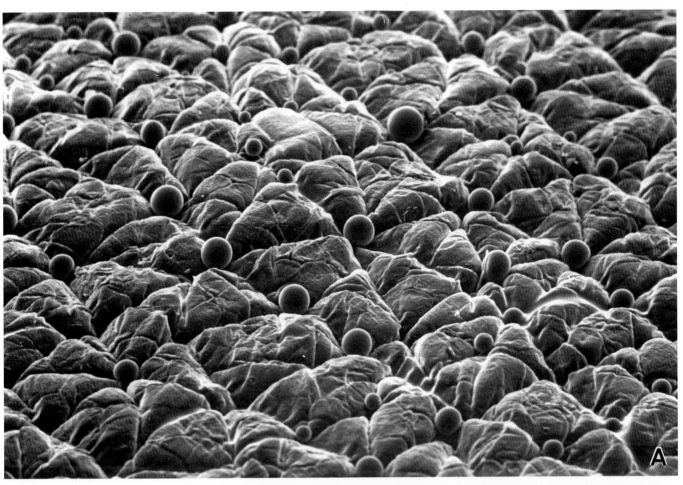

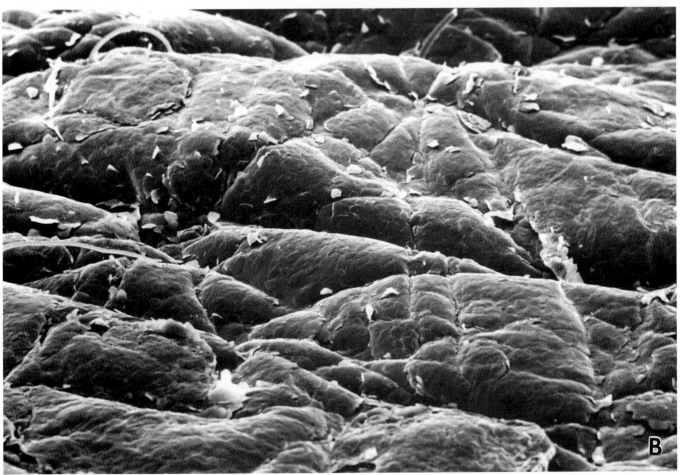

PLATE 5

SKIN TOPOGRAPHY

A. Computer reconstruction of the surface of the calf skin of a 20-year-old woman. This is a very detailed surface with sharp topographic relief. Courtesy of Dr. D. G. Sawermann.

B. As above, from the calf skin of a 35-year-old woman. Although there is only 15 years' difference from Figure A, the skin surface is less detailed. Courtesy of Dr. D. G. Sawermann.

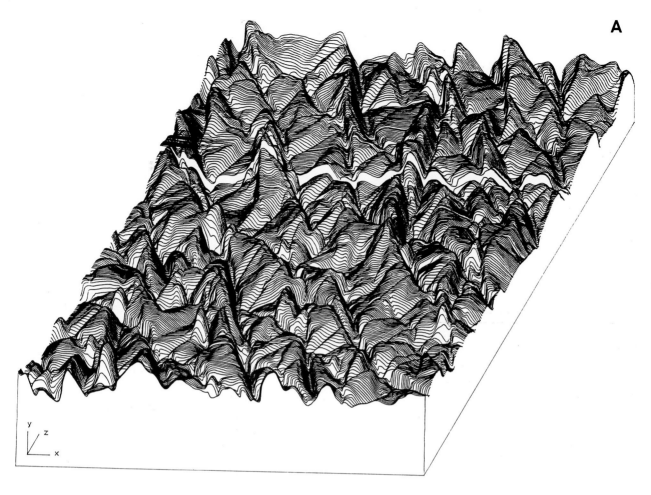

A

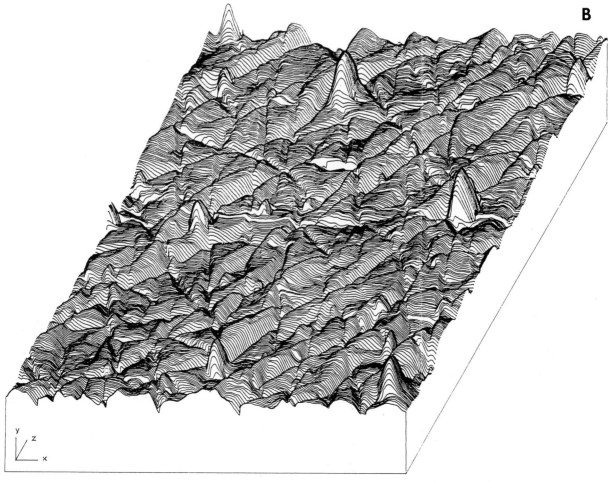

B

PLATE 6

FACIAL SKIN EPIDERMIS

The outer layer of the skin, the epidermis, is a stratified squamous epithelium. The majority of cells are the keratinocytes, which are organized into layers. The layers are named either for their function or their structure. Resident cells interspersed among the keratinocytes may be lymphocytes, Langerhans cells, melanocytes, or Merkel cells.

A. Epidermis from the malar eminence of a 20-year-old White woman who has avoided the sun. Note the shapes of the cells in each layer. The basal keratinocytes (BK) have cytoplasmic rootlets (serrations) that extend into the papillary dermis. In the malpighian layer (ML), the keratinocytes gradually become flattened and aligned parallel to the surface, and develop keratohyalin granules. In the two to three layers of the stratum granulosum (SG), the keratinocytes are stretched horizontally. The stratum lucidum (SL) is compact, and the stratum corneum (SC) appears gelatinous at its base and lacy in its upper part. Melanocytes (M). Langerhans cell (L). 2-μm plastic section. H and Lee. OM 630x.

B. In this epidermis from the malar eminence of a 35-year-old woman, the basal keratinocytes show only a suggestion of cytoplasmic rootlets. The clear delineation of these basal rootlets is an individual characteristic. The stratum corneum (SC) has a basket-weave appearance, an artifact of processing for histology. The actual structure is coherent and without such spaces. Stratum granulosum (SG). Stratum lucidum (SL). Melanocyte (M). Langerhans cell (L). 2-μm plastic section. H and Lee. OM 630x.

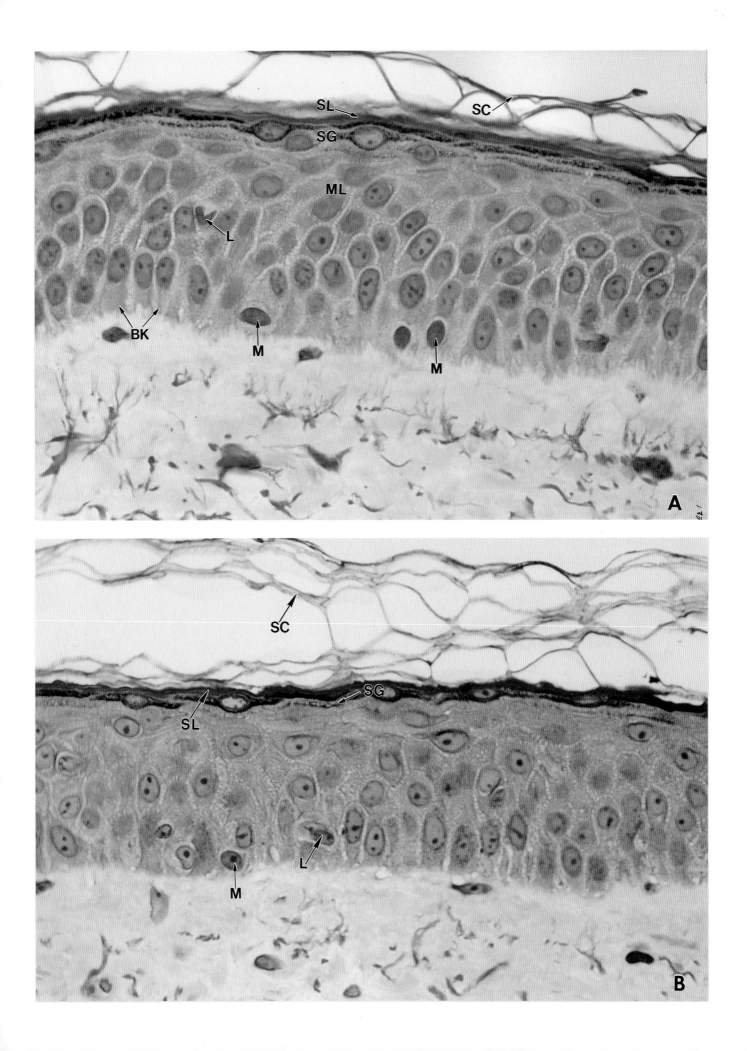

PLATE 7

THICK EPIDERMIS

Volar Surface

There are many regional differences in the structure of the epidermis. One of the most pronounced differences is in its thickness.

A. Stratification in the epidermis from the volar surface of a finger. Note the prominent stratum lucidum (L) and thick stratum corneum (C). The duct of a sweat gland (D) winds through the stratum corneum. Deep rete ridges are characteristic of friction surface epidermis. The corneocytes, the cells of the stratum corneum, and the cells lining the duct of the sweat gland have different staining properties. 2-μm plastic section. H and Lee. OM 160x.

B. The duct of a sweat gland (arrows) weaves its way through thick palmar surface epidermis. 2-μm plastic section. H and Lee. OM 250x.

C. The tight corkscrew pattern of a sweat duct in thick epidermis. The duct is cut several times (arrows) inside an epidermal ridge. 4-μm plastic section. Gridley's reticulin fiber technique. OM 250x.

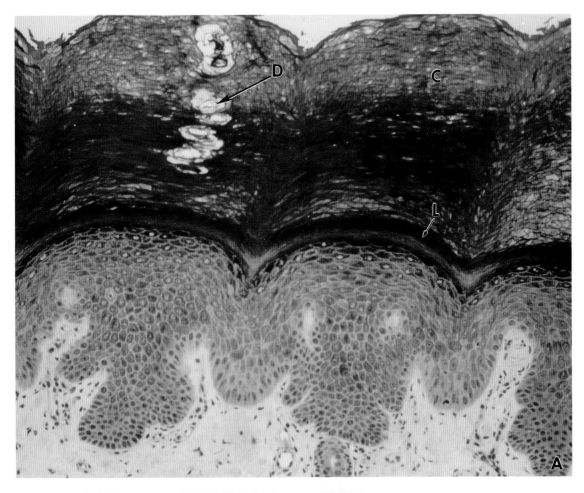

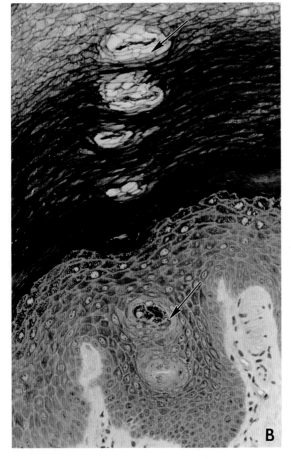

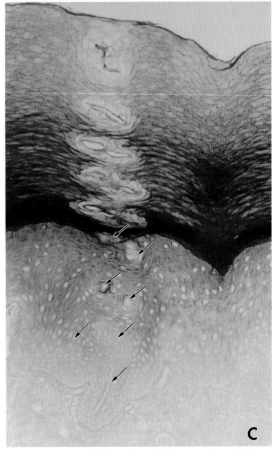

PLATE 8

KERATINIZATION

The epidermis is a self-renewing stratified epithelium composed primarily of keratinocytes. It takes about 1 month from the time a basal cell leaves the bottom layer until it is desquamated. Differentiation is a genetically programmed event that begins with a postmitotic keratinocyte and terminates with a nonviable cell. The events of cell differentiation include:

1. Synthesis and modification of structural proteins, especially keratins
2. Appearance of new organelles, reorganization of existing organelles, and loss of organelles
3. Change in cell size and shape
4. Specialization of cellular metabolism
5. Changes in the properties of cell membranes
6. Dehydration

The keratinocytes are organized into various layers that represent different stages of differentiation, as illustrated in this schematic diagram.

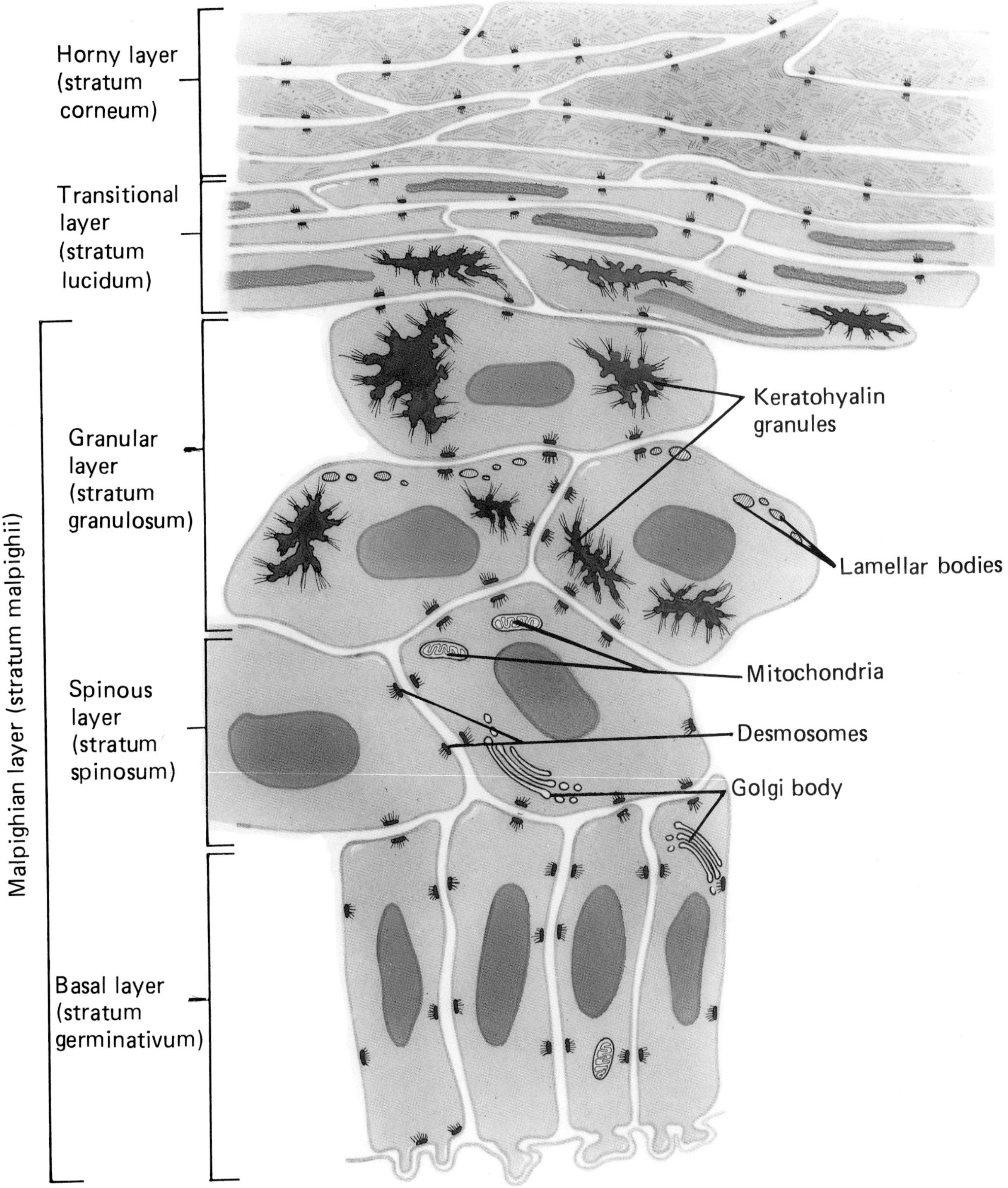

Horny layer
(stratum
corneum)

Transitional
layer
(stratum
lucidum)

Granular
layer
(stratum
granulosum)

Spinous
layer
(stratum
spinosum)

Basal layer
(stratum
germinativum)

Malpighian layer (stratum malpighii)

Keratohyalin
granules

Lamellar bodies

Mitochondria

Desmosomes

Golgi body

PLATE 9

EPIDERMAL KERATIN

The family of keratins consists of more than 20 different polypeptides. The particular species of keratins in an epidermal keratinocyte depend on its location in the epidermis and its state of differentiation. Basal cells contain only the lower-molecular-weight keratins, which are associated with proliferation; as keratinocytes differentiate in the malpighian layer, they produce more higher-molecular-weight keratins.

A. The distribution of the keratin fibers that make up the cytoskeleton of human keratinocytes is shown by indirect immunofluorescence, using a polyclonal antibody against keratins. OM 800x. Courtesy of Dr. R. R. Sun.

B. Enlarged, colored photograph of keratin fibers using the same treatment as in Figure A. The bundles of keratin filaments make up the structural backbone of epidermal cells and give them stability. OM 1000x. Courtesy of Dr. R. R. Sun.

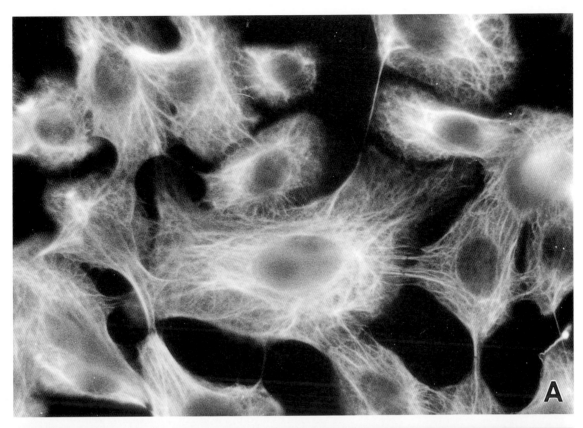

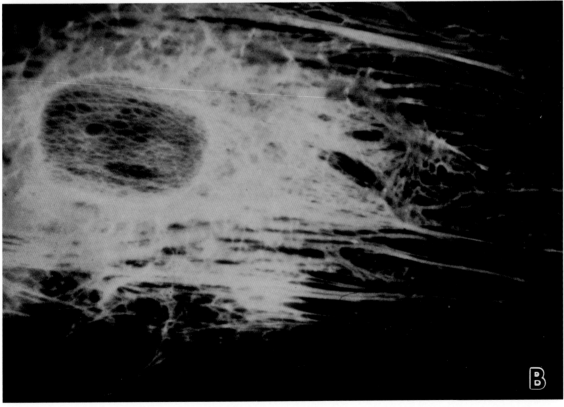

PLATE 10

EPIDERMAL LAYERS

The keratinocytes of the epidermis are divided into layers:

1. Basal layer or stratum germinativum
2. Spinous layer or stratum spinosum
3. Granular layer or stratum granulosum
4. Transitional layer or stratum lucidum
5. Horny layer or stratum corneum

A. The granular layer (G) is named for its cells, which contain basophilic granules when seen under the light microscope; the granules contain keratohyalin. Above this layer is the compact stratum lucidum (SL). The horny layer or stratum corneum (C) is the superficial dead layer of the epidermis; it is the major barrier of the skin. Flattened corneocytes make up the stratum corneum. From the facial skin of a young woman. 2-μm plastic section. H and Lee. OM 630x.

B. The keratinocytes in the spinous layer are named for the spine-like appearance that results from shrinking during the processing of the tissues. "Spines" have been shown with the TEM to contain attachment plaques, or desmosomes, within the intercellular space (IS). Spinous cells have keratin filaments, also known as tonofilaments, in their cytoplasm. From the facial skin. 2-μm plastic section. H and Lee. OM 630x.

C. The basal keratinocytes give rise to cells that move up to the more superficial layers. The basal layer in this photograph also contains clear cells, which are pigment-forming melanocytes (M), and a Langerhans cell (L), which is probably migrating into, or out of, the epidermis. Both of these cells have smooth borders and do not form intercellular bridges with adjacent cells. Papillary dermis (PD). 2-μm plastic section. H and Lee. OM 630x.

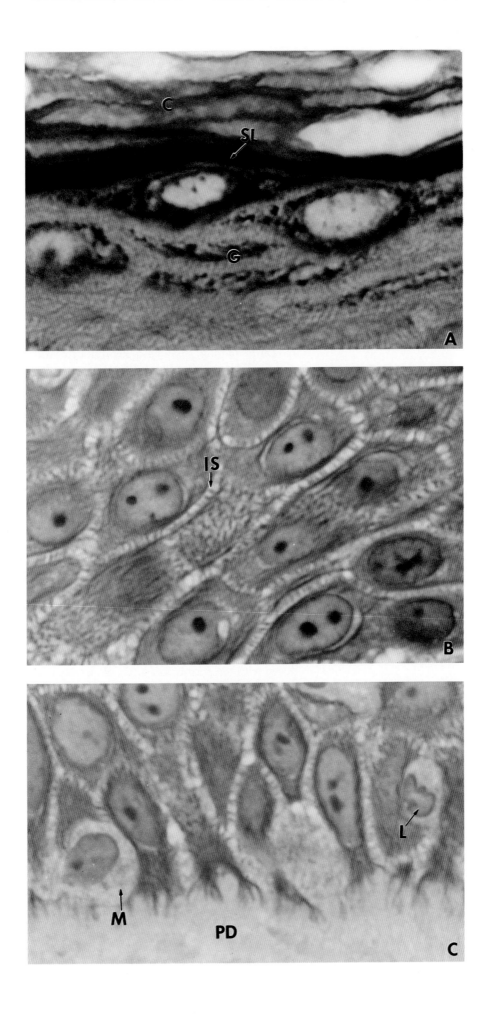

PLATE 11

BASAL KERATINOCYTES

The basal layer is a heterogeneous mixture of cells. Some basal keratinocytes divide and give rise to differentiating keratinocytes. Other basal keratinocytes function as the anchoring cells.

A. Dark-staining, small basal keratinocytes with short, or no, cytoplasmic footlets, found at the bases of rete ridges, are the epidermal stem cells. These are relatively undifferentiated, slowly cycling cells that are available on demand. These cells divide and give rise to two daughter cells each. One remains behind as a stem cell, and the other becomes an "amplifying" cell that divides rapidly and finally differentiates into a corneocyte. The presence of stem cells shows that there is a highly ordered self-renewing mechanism in the epidermis. Papillary dermis (PD). 1-μm plastic section. Toluidine blue. OM 630x. Reproduced with the permission of Dr. R. Lavker, Epidermal Stem Cells, *Journal of Investigative Dermatology* 81:123s, © by Williams & Wilkins, 1983.

B. Some basal cells, mainly distributed along the sides of rete ridges, are specialized for anchoring the epidermis onto the dermal surface; they have a limited capacity to divide and differentiate into corneocytes. These basal keratinocytes have conspicuous cytoplasmic extensions or serrations (arrows) and many tonofilaments (once known as Herxheimer filaments) in their cytoplasm. Papillary dermis (PD). 1-μm plastic section. Toluidine blue. OM 630x. Reproduced with the permission of Dr. R. Lavker, Epidermal Stem Cells, *Journal of Investigative Dermatology* 81:123s, © by Williams & Wilkins, 1983.

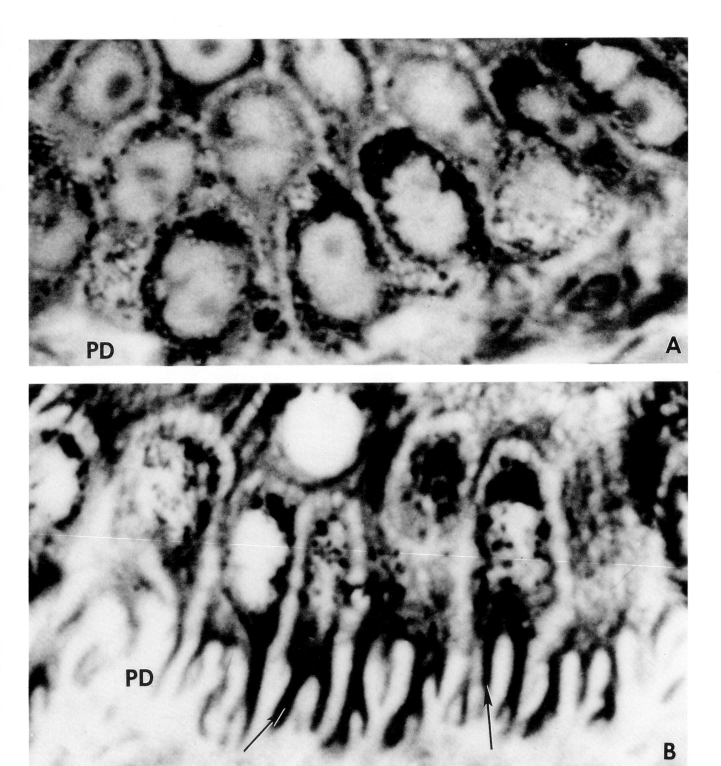

PLATE 12

BASAL KERATINOCYTES

A. This epidermis from the chin of a middle-aged man has rete ridges with a heterogeneous population of basal keratinocytes. The cells at the base of the ridges are smaller than those at the sides and in the arcades that connect the ridges. The keratinocytes at the sides of the rete (arrow) and those of the arcades have distinct cytoplasmic rootlets (serrations); these are thought to be the anchoring cells of the epidermis. The keratinocytes at the base (arrowheads) of the ridges have practically no rootlets; these are thought to be stem cells. There are many melanocytes (M) interspersed among the basal keratinocytes. 2-μm plastic section. H and Lee. OM 250x.

B. Mitosis occurs in the basal or suprabasal cells at the tips of the ridges. A higher magnification of the base of one of the ridges, in the same section as in Figure A, shows two dividing suprabasal cells that may have arisen from a stem cell (arrow). Stem cells have a high nuclear/cytoplasmic ratio. Melanocyte (M). 2-μm plastic section. H and Lee. OM 1000x.

C. This epidermal ridge from the same skin as in Figures A and B shows the basal cells (arrowheads) with small or no cytoplasmic rootlets, typical of stem cells. The sides consist of cells with cytoplasmic extensions (arrows) characteristic of anchoring cells. 4-μm plastic section. Gridley's reticulin fiber technique. OM 1000x.

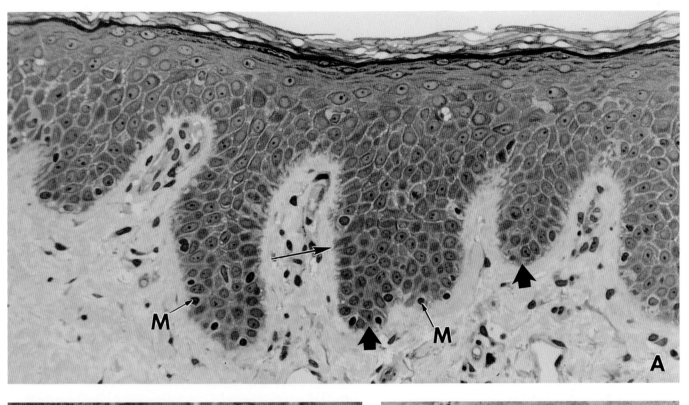

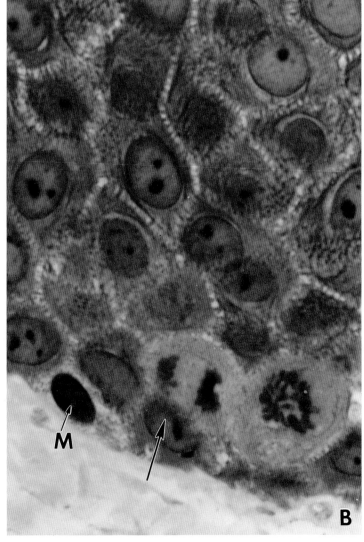

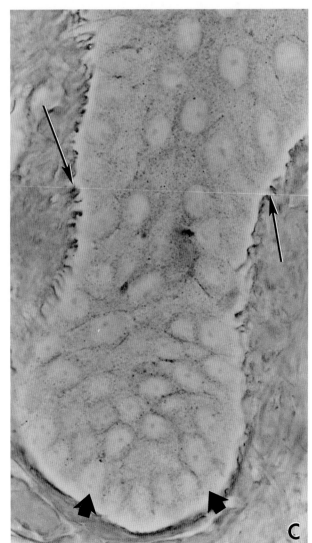

PLATE 13

EPIDERMIS

Mitosis

The epidermis is in a steady state of cell production and cell loss. Mitotically active cells in the basal layers move upward, differentiate, and die. In order for the epidermis to maintain a constant thickness, the number of proliferating and differentiated cells has to be regulated. The dermis, hormones, vitamin A and its derivatives, epidermal growth factor, and cyclic nucleotides are some of the factors that participate in this regulation.

All the mitotic figures in this plate are from the epidermis of facial skin of middle-aged White women. 2-μm plastic sections. H and Lee. OM 1000x.

A. Two mitotic figures: prophase (P) in the suprabasal layer and anaphase (A) in the basal layer of the epidermis. One daughter cell from each mitotic figure will leave the lower layer and differentiate into a corneocyte.

B. Metaphase (M) in the basal layer (possibly a stem cell) next to a melanocyte (Me).

C. Mitotic figures in suprabasal cells: the one on the left is in telophase (T) and the one on the right is in metaphase (M).

D. Early anaphase (A) in a suprabasal keratinocyte. Note that some chromosomes appear to be lagging.

E. Late anaphase (A) in the basal layer.

F. Suprabasal telophase (T) in the process of forming two daughter cells.

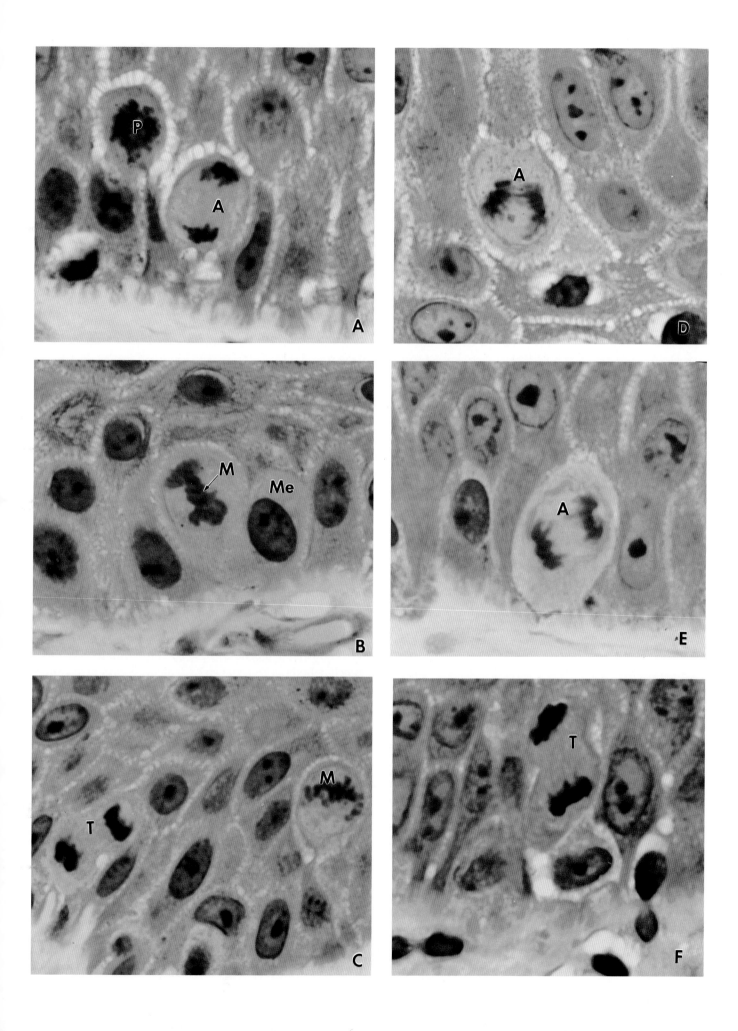

PLATE 14

LOWER EPIDERMIS, DESMOSOME, LAMELLAR BODY

A. TEM micrograph of basal keratinocytes with bundles of keratin filaments (F) and melanosomes (M) in their cytoplasm. These structures surround the nucleus (N). The keratinocytes rest on the basal lamina (BL). From the face of a young Black woman. OM 3200x.

B. Higher magnification of a keratinocyte, in the lower epidermis, which contains clusters of filaments (F) and membrane-bound melanosomes (M). Keratinocytes are rich in biosynthetic organelles; mitochondria (Mi) provide the needed energy. Desmosomes (D) join adjacent keratinocytes. Basal lamina (BL). From the face of a young Black woman. OM 13,000x.

C. TEM micrograph of desmosomes (D) from the spinous layer. Desmosomes are junctions in the intercellular space (IC) that join adjacent keratinocytes and serve as anchoring plates for keratin filaments. The intercellular space between epidermal cells represents an extension of the extracellular compartment of the dermis to the stratum corneum. This space permits nutrients from the dermal blood vessels to perfuse the nonvascular epidermis and the secretory products of the epidermis to reach the dermis. OM 25,000x. Courtesy of Prof. R.A.J. Eady.

D. TEM micrograph of membrane-bound granules with alternating lamellae, known as lamellar bodies (L). The primary site of action of lamellar bodies, also known as Odland bodies or membrane-coating granules, is at the transition of the upper granular and the cornified layers. They fuse with the cell membrane and release their contents into the intercellular space. They contain acid hydrolases and may act as lysosomes. These organelles first appear in the upper spinous layer and persist up to the junction of the granular and horny layers. Melanosome (M). Desmosome (D). From the face of a young Black woman. OM 40,000x. Courtesy of Michael Webb.

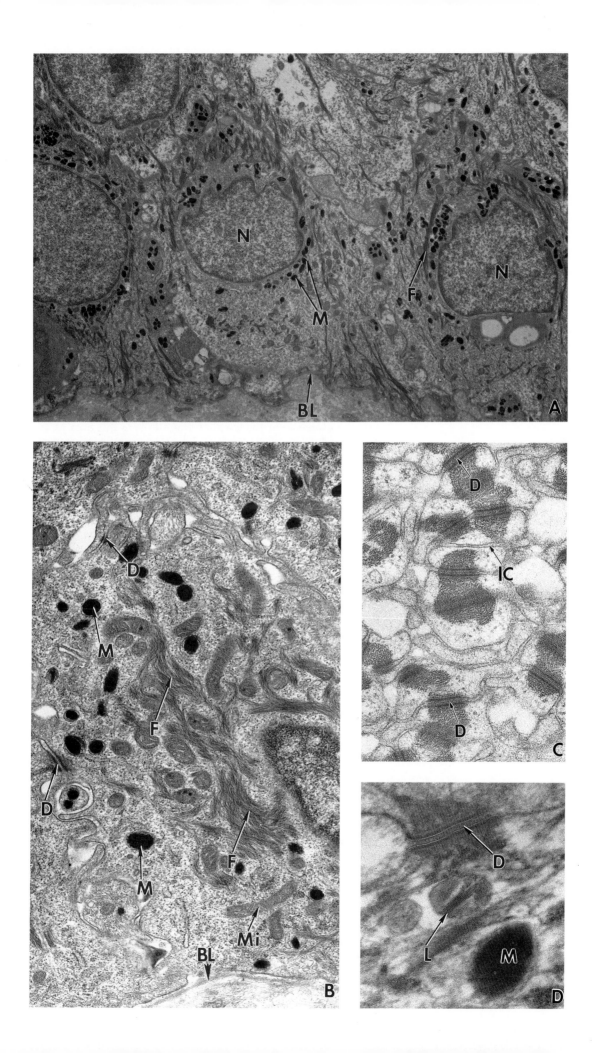

PLATE 15

UPPER EPIDERMAL LAYERS

A. TEM micrograph showing the transitional area between the stratum granulosum (G) and the stratum lucidum (L). The granular cells and their keratohyalin granules (K) play a decisive role in the programmed transformation of a keratinocyte to a cornified cell. The viable granular cell differentiates into a nonviable corneocyte; this change involves the loss of the nucleus and most of the organelles, with the exception of the keratin filaments and the matrix material. Many enzymes are involved in the degradation. The main site of action of the lamellar granules is in this area. A transitional cell (T) has a highly heterochromatic nucleus, is electron-dense, and contains few recognizable organelles. OM 8100x.

B. Keratohyalin granules (K) are in the granular cells; the keratohyalin granules correspond to the basophilic granules seen with the light microscope. Keratohyalin is made up of a precursor form of the protein filaggrin. Conversion of the filaggrin precursor to the product occurs during the transition of a granular cell to a cornified cell. Desmosomes may remain between cells. Stratum corneum (C), stratum lucidum (L). OM 25,000x. Courtesy of Dr. Mary Bell.

C. TEM micrograph of the upper epidermis: stratum granulosum, stratum lucidum (L), and stratum corneum (C). The transition from a granular cell to a horny, or cornified cell involves a 50 to 85% loss in dry weight of the cell. Keratins account for 80% of the cornified cell. Horny cells are flattened; they provide the major barrier of the skin. Keratohyalin granule (K). Lamellar granule (G). OM 15,000x. Courtesy of Dr. Mary Bell.

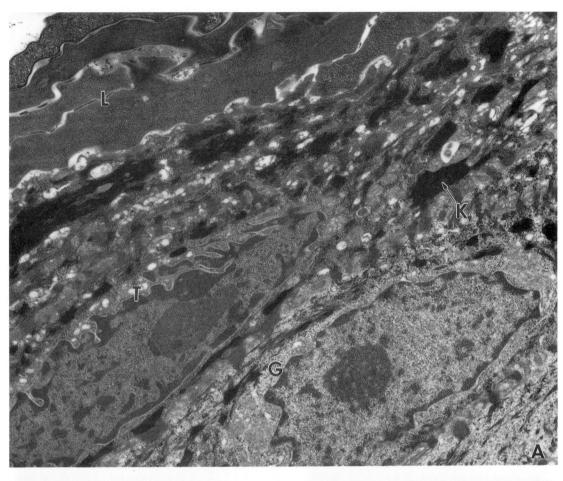

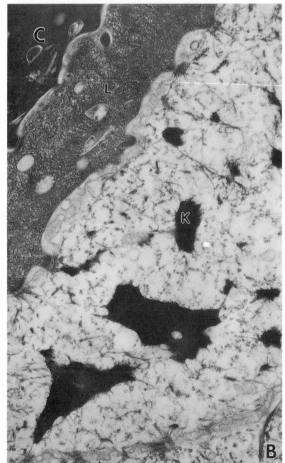

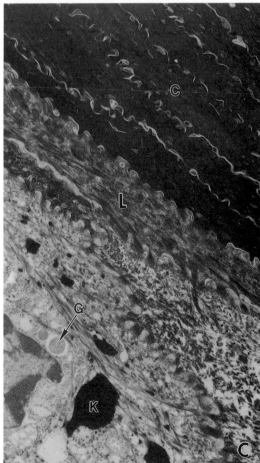

PLATE 16

STRATUM GRANULOSUM and STRATUM LUCIDUM

Keratinocytes undergo biochemical and structural changes during differentiation. These changes include fluctuations in water content, keratin species, numerous enzymes, filaggrin, and involucrin. Changes in structural and biochemical components may account for different staining properties of the keratinocytes.

A. Epidermis from the back of the hand showing the red-stained stratum lucidum immediately below the horny layer. Regardless of body region, all epidermis has a stratum lucidum. 1-μm plastic section. Toluidine blue and basic fuchsin. OM 400x.

B. The cells of the stratum granulosum (G) and stratum lucidum (L) stain with picrosirius red, a stain that is normally used to demonstrate collagenous fibers. This is the epidermis from the face of a young White woman. 2-μm plastic section. Picrosirius red, pH 2.0. OM 400x.

C. The keratohyalin granules (K) in the stratum granulosum stain with colloidal iron techniques for mucopolysaccharides. The keratohyalin granules may contain a mucopolysaccharide in addition to the proteins known to occur in them. In the stratum lucidum (L), only the material inside the two vesicles (arrows) stains with the Hale technique, but this is probably an artifact. 2-μm plastic section. Hale's colloidal iron technique, pH 1.0, lightly counterstained with nuclear fast red. OM 1200x.

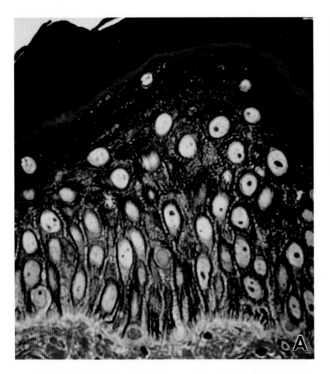

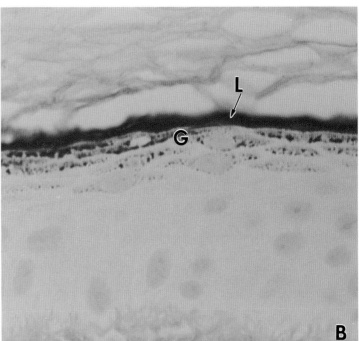

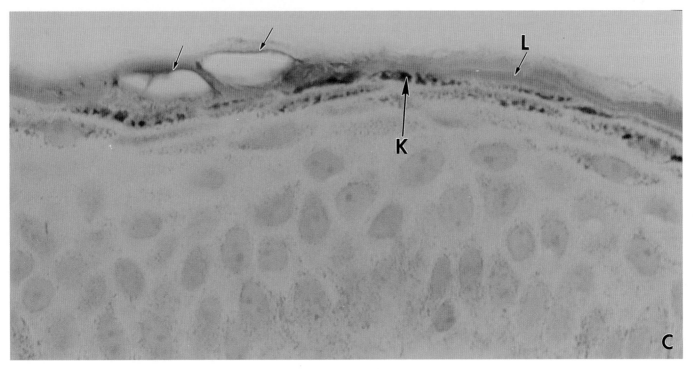

PLATE 17

UPPER EPIDERMIS

A. Stratum granulosum (SG) and stratum lucidum (SL) from the finger of a 36-year-old man. The jagged keratohyalin granules tend to fuse as the keratinocytes rise to the stratum lucidum. The transition from a viable to a nonviable cell occurs when the keratinocyte changes from a granular cell to a stratum lucidum cell. Several enzymes have been shown to participate in the degradation of the viable keratinocyte. 2-μm plastic section. H and Lee. OM 1200x.

B. These corneocytes, from the finger of a child, are closely cemented together by a dark-staining material that may correspond to the precursor protein, involucrin, which forms a sturdy envelope around the cell. The stratum corneum is the major barrier of the skin. Acidic and basic keratins make up about 80% of the dry mass of the corneocytes. 2-μm plastic section. H and Lee. OM 800x.

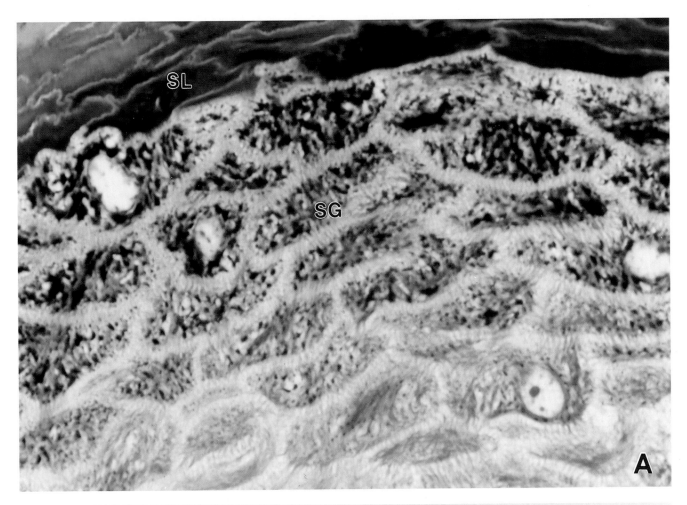

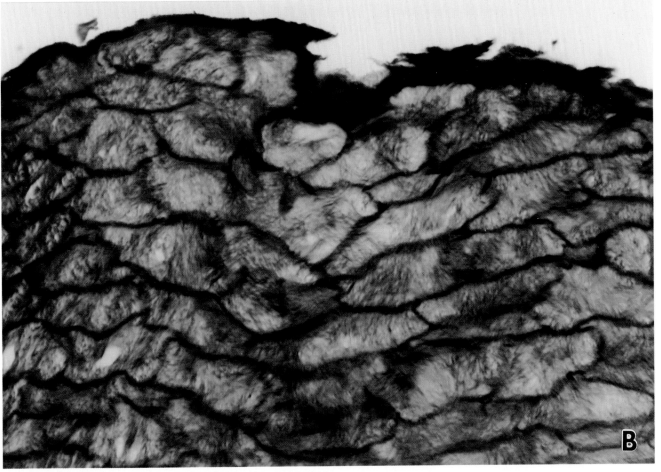

PLATE 18

THICK EPIDERMIS
Stratum Granulosum

A. The keratohyalin granules (K) in the stratum granulosum and the stratum lucidum (L) of the volar surface of the finger stain with a mixture of sirius red and sirius blue, pH 2.0. The granules are dispersed, metabolized, and become invisible in the stratum corneum (C). 2-μm plastic section. OM 800x.

B. The keratohyalin granules (arrow) stain with the colloidal iron technique. This indicates that these histidine-rich filaggrin precursor granules may contain mucopolysaccharides. From the finger epidermis of a 36-year-old man. 2-μm plastic section. Hale's colloidal iron technique, pH 1.0. OM 800x.

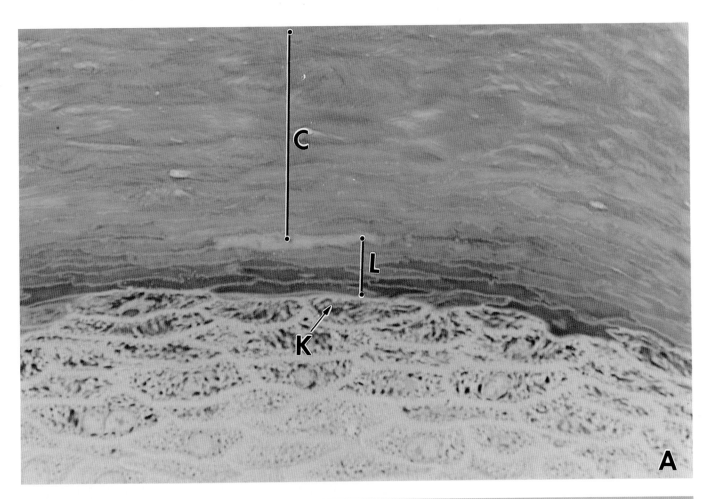

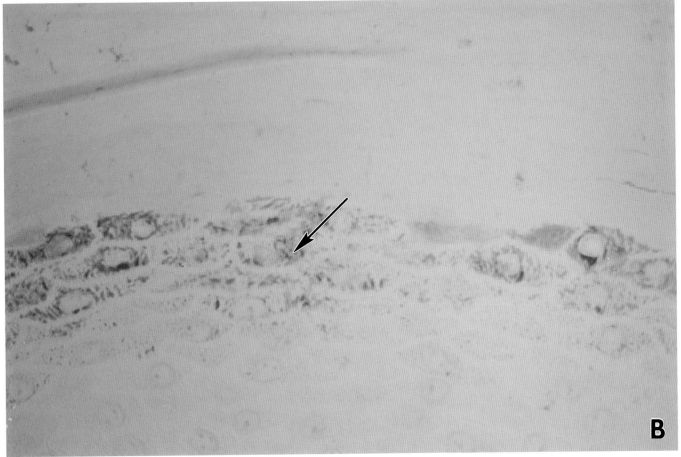

PLATE 19

KERATOHYALIN GRANULES and LAMELLAR GRANULES

Immunofluorescence is a powerful tool for precise localization of specific biochemical markers.

A. Double immunofluorescence staining in a frozen section of abdominal skin treated with the monoclonal antibody AE17 to lamellar granules, also called Odland bodies. AE17 antibody recognizes the 25K protein in lamellar granules. These granules fuse with the cell membranes between the upper granular and the lower cornified cell layers, discharge their contents into the intercellular spaces, and become rearranged in lamellar arrays. OM 375x. Courtesy of Dr. T. T. Sun.

B. Double immunofluorescence staining in a frozen section of abdominal skin treated with a polyclonal antibody to filaggrin. The precursor to filaggrin is a major component of keratohyalin granules. OM 375x. Courtesy of Dr. T. T. Sun.

C. Double immunofluorescence staining in a frozen section of plantar skin treated with the monoclonal antibody AE17 to lamellar granules. The expanded granular cell compartment in this thick epidermis shows the layers of AE 17-positive lamellar granules. OM 375x. Courtesy of Dr. T. T. Sun.

D. Double immunofluorescence staining in a frozen section of plantar skin treated with a polyclonal antibody to filaggrin. This photograph shows the expanded granular cell layer in thick epidermis. Based on keratin data, there is evidence that plantar epidermis differs from trunk epidermis. OM 375x. Courtesy of Dr. T. T. Sun.

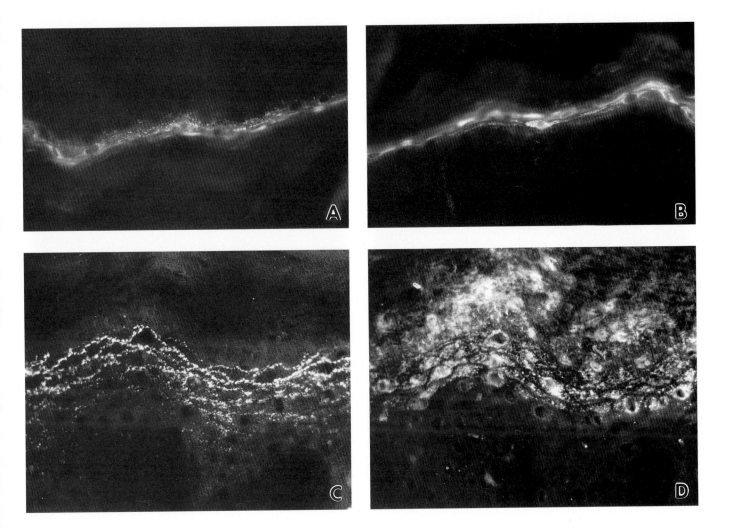

PLATE 20

CORNEOCYTES

The mission of the epidermis is to form the stratum corneum, the protective layer of dead cells that covers the surface. The stratum corneum is an effective barrier to water loss and is mostly impermeable to external substances, which include drugs as well as toxic materials.

A. This SEM micrograph of a small fold on the ankle of a 45-year-old man shows corneocytes flaking off the surface epidermis. The stratum corneum (arrows) is about one-fifth the thickness of the epidermis (E). The papillary dermis (P) consists of small collagenous fiber bundles. OM 120x.

B. SEM micrograph of the surface of the horny layer. The dry, superficial corneocytes are becoming detached. OM 1000x. Reprinted by permission of VCH Publishers, Inc., 220 East 23rd St., New York, NY, 10010 from: Wilborn, Hyde and Montes, *SEM of Normal and Abnormal Human Skin*, p. 74. 1985.

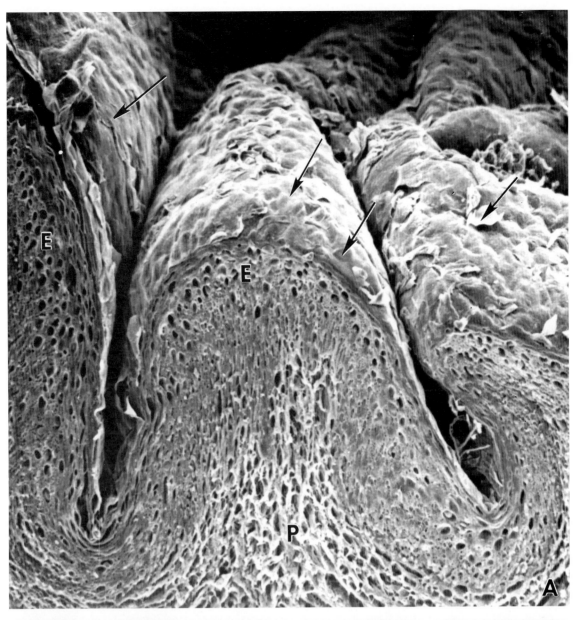

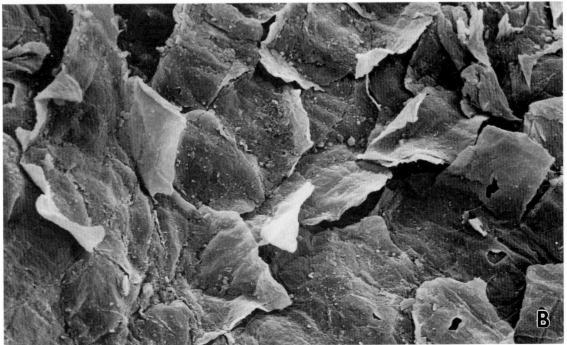

PLATE 21

CORNEOCYTES

A. Surface SEM view of polyhedral corneocytes in flank skin. The thin, flat "squamae" (corneocytes) overlap at their borders. OM 1000x. Courtesy of Dr. Peter Goodkin.

B. SEM micrograph of a corneocyte with a relatively smooth surface. Corneocytes from different regions have distinctive surface topographies, sizes, and shapes, according to functional needs. OM 1000x. Courtesy of Dr. J. L. Laveque.

C. SEM micrograph of the surface of a corneocyte covered with microvilli. Corneocytes interlock with cells in the layers above and below by ridges and villi; this arrangement ensures tight bonding. OM 1000x. Courtesy of Dr. J. L. Laveque.

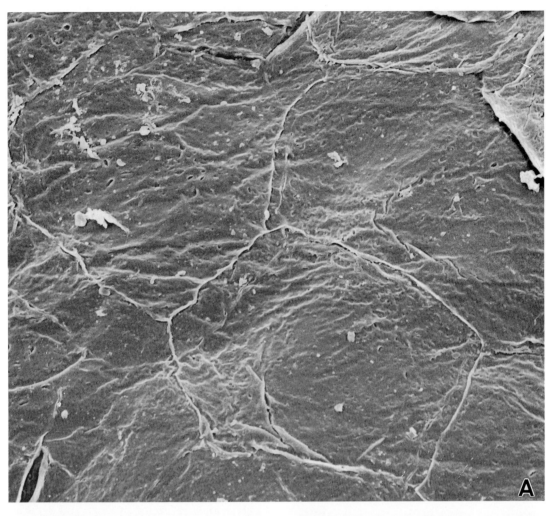

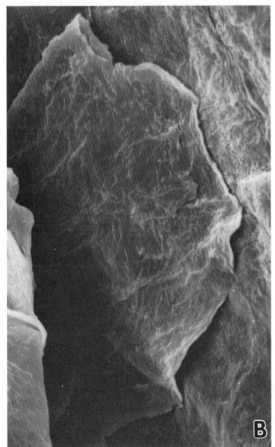

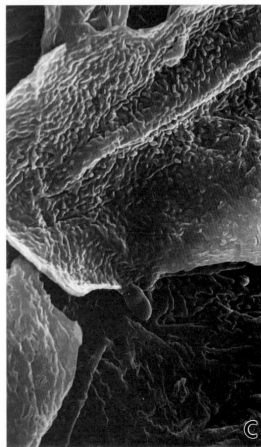

PLATE 22

EPIDERMAL INQUILINE CELLS

The epidermis consists of a mixed population of cell types. Interspersed among the keratinocytes are nonkeratinizing (inquiline) cells that migrate into the epidermis during fetal and postnatal life. The principal immigrant cells include the melanocytes, Langerhans cells, and lymphocytes. Merkel cells are also found in the epidermis.

A. The epidermis is an open door to several types of cells in the dermis. In this epidermis from the face of a White woman, there are several lymphocytes (L) in the basal layer. Lymphocytes play a central role in the immune response. 2-μm plastic section. H and Lee. OM 1000x.

B. Melanocytes or melanin-synthesizing cells are interspersed among the basal keratinocytes and appear as clear cells. In this epidermis from the face of a young Black woman, the melanocytes (M) have a pale cytoplasm, round nucleus, and dendrites (arrows) that extend between the keratinocytes. 2-μm plastic section. H and Lee. OM 1000x.

C. Langerhans cells (L) are present in the spinous layer; the cells can be identified with moderate certainty with the light microscope by their pale cytoplasm, convoluted nucleus, and the absence of both tonofilaments and intercellular spines at their periphery. They are derived from the bone marrow and are the prime movers of the skin's immunological functions. A mast cell (Ma) is located near a blood vessel (BV). From the face of a 34-year-old man. Melanocyte (M). 2-μm plastic section. H and Lee. OM 1000x.

D. Langerhans cell (L) in the upper malpighian layer of the epidermis of a 59-year-old man. Early in development and throughout postnatal life, Langerhans cells migrate from the dermis into the epidermis, and vice versa, especially during allergic reactions. 2-μm plastic section. H and Lee. OM 1000x.

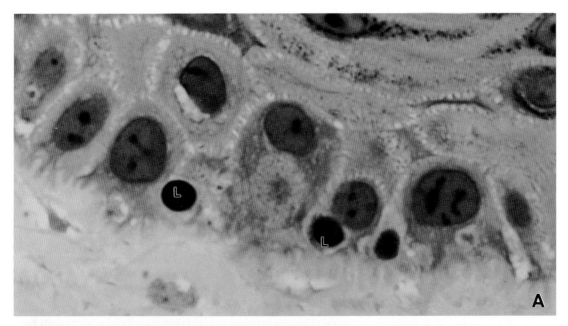

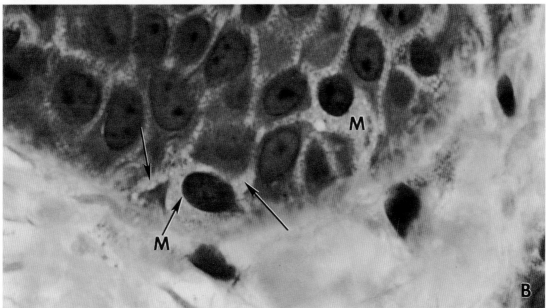

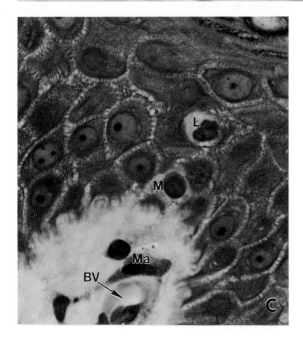

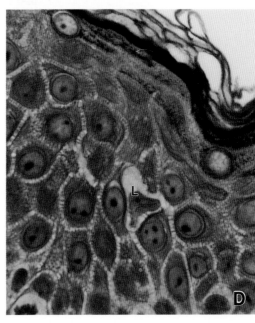

PLATE 23

EPIDERMAL MELANOCYTES

Melanocytes, which are derived from the neural crest, are interspersed among basal cells and interact with a specific number of keratinocytes in the "epidermal melanocyte unit."

A. Dendritic melanocytes have invaded the vermilion border of the lower lip in an 8-month fetus. Silver impregnation indicates the presence of melanin pigment granules. 30-μm frozen section. Winkelmann's silver impregnation method. OM 20x.

B. Highly branched melanocytes between the epidermis (E) and the mesenchyme (M) at the cutaneous border of the lip of an 8-month fetus. From the same section as Figure A. OM 40x.

C. Schema of an epidermal melanocyte unit showing a melanocyte and its constellation of about 36 keratinocytes. Melanosomes are synthesized in the Golgi system (G) of melanocytes and are distributed to the surrounding keratinocytes by the dendrites (D). The keratinocytes transport and degrade the melanin. The transfer of pigment may take place either by the fusion and breakdown of the membranes of both the melanocyte and the keratinocyte, or by the phagocytosis of the tips of the pigment-containing melanocyte dendrites by the keratinocyte. The transfer of melanin from a melanocyte dendrite to a keratinocyte was hypothesized by Masson to be like the injection of substances with a syringe (cytocrine). Epidermal melanocytes divide at a rate that keeps pace with the turnover of keratinocytes. Courtesy of Dr. W. Quevedo, Jr. adapted from T. B. Fitzpatrick and A. S. Breathnach. Reproduced with permission from *American Zoologist*, 9:532, 1969.

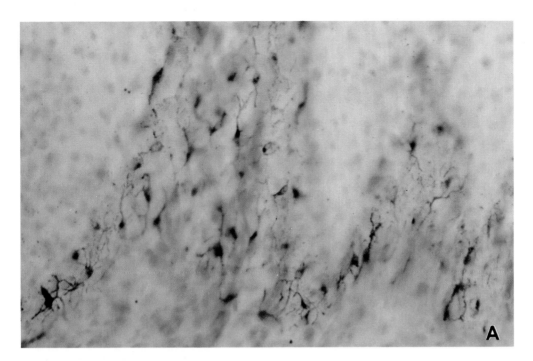

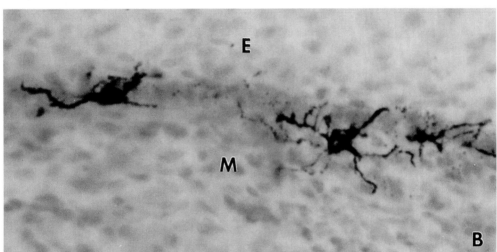

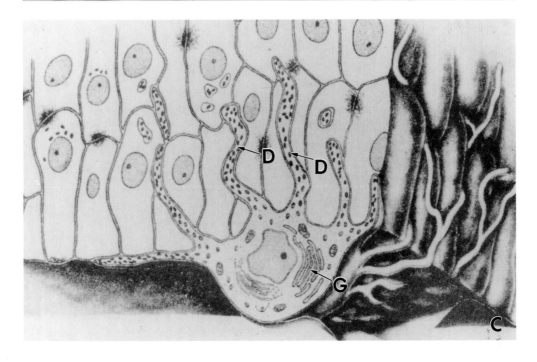

PLATE 24

MELANOCYTE

Generally, the melanocytes in sun-exposed epidermis are larger and have more dendrites than those in the epidermis of sun-protected skin. However, if covered skin is exposed to ultraviolet light, the melanocytes increase in size and their dendrites branch. The darkness of skin color is dependent more on melanocyte activity than on the number of melanocytes. Melanocytes are confined to the basal layer, or they hang like a pendant from the epidermis, as seen in this TEM micrograph from the hand of a 65-year-old man. A large, pendulous melanocyte (PM) appears to hang from the epidermis. There are no keratin fibrils in the cytoplasm of melanocytes, and hemidesmosomes and desmosomes are not seen on the peripheral cell membranes. Another melanocyte (M) resides in the basal layer; it is surrounded by keratinocytes (K) with their characteristic tonofilaments. Papillary dermis (PD). OM 3200x.

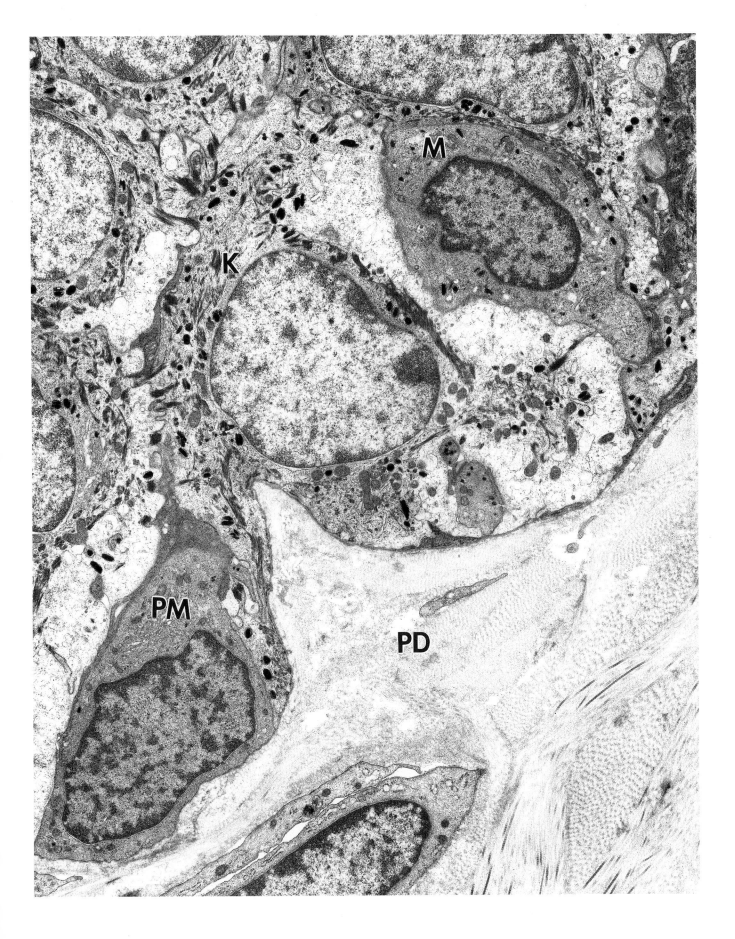

PLATE 25

MELANOCYTE

A. TEM micrograph of an epidermal melanocyte containing melanosomes (M) in different stages of development. All melanosomes are membrane-bound and have the same specific enzyme, tyrosinase. Melanosomes are categorized into four developmental stages according to their fine structure. Nucleus (N). Golgi body (G). Nearby keratinocytes (K) are recognized by their keratin filaments. OM 13,000x.

B. Stage I melanosomes (arrows) are mainly oval, membrane-bound vesicles that contain sparse filaments with a periodicity of 9 to 10 nm. OM 37,000x.

C. Stage II melanosomes (arrow) are oval bodies that contain membranous filaments, often crosslinked, with a periodicity of 9 to 10 nm. OM 37,000x.

D. Stage III melanosomes (arrow) are like those in stage II, but melanin partially obscures their internal structure. OM 37,000x.

E. Stage IV melanosomes (arrow) are oval bodies in which melanin completely obscures the internal filamentous structure seen in stages II and III. OM 37,000x.

Figures A, B, C, D, and E courtesy of Dr. F. Hu. From Melanocyte Cytology in Normal Skin, Melanocytic Nevi and Malignant Melanosomes, *Masson Monographs in Dermatopathology, Vol. 1*, reproduced with permission of Masson Publications. 1981.

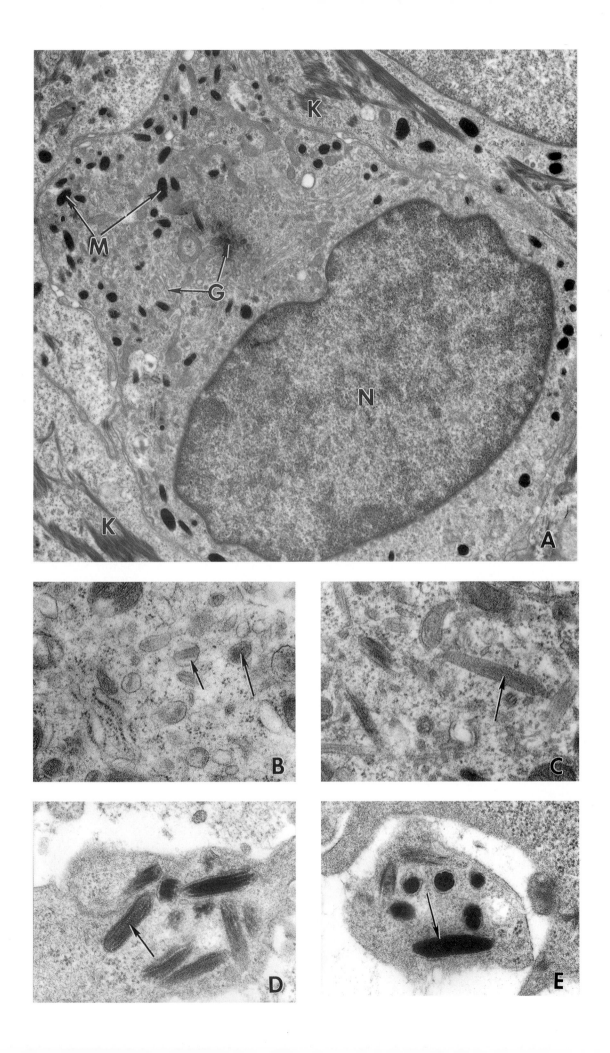

PLATE 26

KERATINOCYTES
Melanosomes

The color of the skin is related to the size, number, and distribution of melanosomes; color depends upon the pigment in melanosomes and not the density of melanocytes. More pigment is present in the lower epidermal layers than in the superficial layers.

A. Sparse argyrophilic melanosomes in the photodamaged facial skin of a young blonde woman. Some basal or suprabasal keratinocytes (arrows) contain granules that stain brownish-yellow rather than black with ammoniacal silver nitrate; such staining may indicate different types of melanin or immature melanosomes. Photodamage may also adversely affect the formation of normal melanosomes. 2-μm plastic section. Fontana-Masson silver technique counterstained with H and Lee. OM 200x.

B. Facial skin epidermis from a brunette White woman. There are many argyrophilic melanosomes in all layers of the epidermis, including some in the horny layer. Melanin protects the skin by absorbing and scattering radiation. 2-μm plastic section. Fontana-Masson silver technique counterstained with H and Lee. OM 250x.

C. Facial skin of a dark-skinned young White woman. There are many melanosomes in all the epidermal layers. In the basal layers, the melanosomes tend to gather above the nucleus (arrow), a mechanism that may protect the vulnerable DNA from potentially harmful ultraviolet radiation. Melanocyte (M). 2-μm plastic section. Fontana-Masson silver technique counterstained with nuclear fast red. OM 250x.

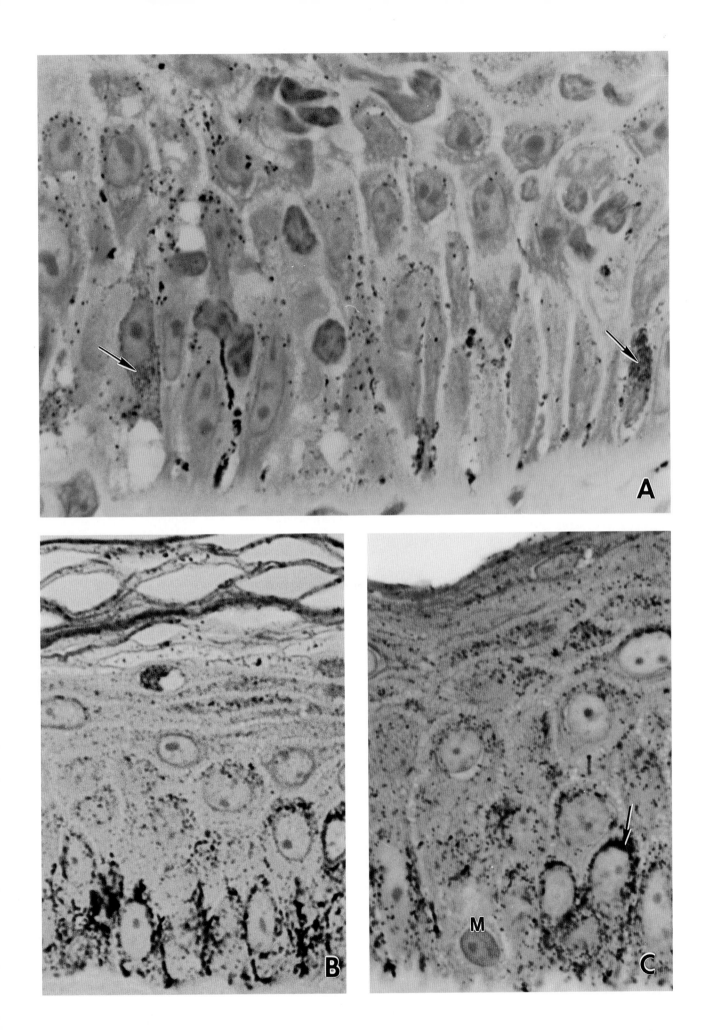

PLATE 27

KERATINOCYTES

Melanosomes

The number of melanocytes is the same in all races; however, melanocytes of darkly pigmented skin have thicker, longer, branched dendrites. The differences in pigmentation depend upon the quantity of melanin produced and the distribution of pigment granules.

A. Heavy concentration of melanosomes in the epidermis of the face of a young Black African woman. The melanosomes tend to form supranuclear caps on the basal keratinocytes. Melanosomes may remain in all layers of the epidermis in Black skin; they are degraded by lysosomal enzymes as keratinization occurs, but they are not as completely degraded in Black skin as in White skin. 2-μm plastic section. Fontana-Masson silver technique. OM 500x.

B. Individual melanosomes inside corneocytes in the horny layer and in the keratinocytes of the upper malpighian layer of the facial epidermis of a young Black woman. 2-μm plastic section. Fontana-Masson silver technique. OM 1000x.

C. Numerous melanosomes form supranuclear caps in the basal layer of this epidermis from the trunk skin of a young Black woman. Pendulous melanocytes (PM), cells that hang from the epidermis, occur more often in dark than in light skin. 2-μm plastic section. Fontana-Masson silver technique counterstained with fast green. OM 1000x.

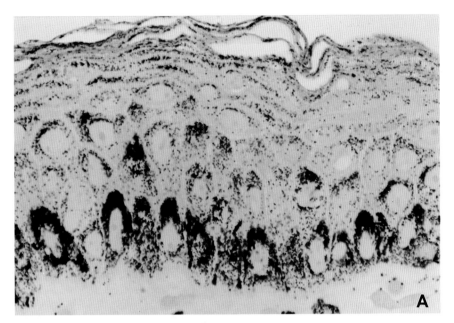

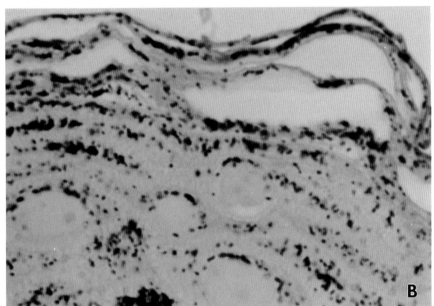

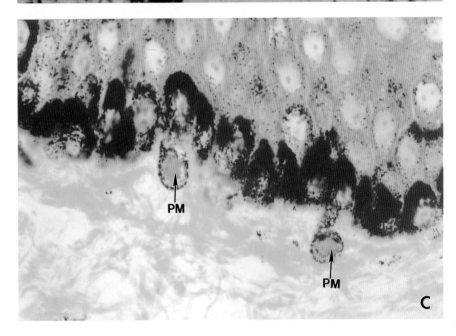

PLATE 28

KERATINOCYTES

Melanosomes

These 2 μ plastic sections were stained with the Fontana-Masson technique. The microscopic images were captured with a Sony CCD camera and processed in a Zeiss IBAS 2000 image analyser. Three regions of the skin (basal epidermis, mid and upper epidermis, and the papillary dermis) were interactively excised from the image and the pigment was converted to binary image form by grey-level segmentation. The three resultant images were copied into the original image at specific grey levels to which selected colors (basal layer: blue; mid and upper epidermis: red; papillary dermis: green) were assigned.

A. Epidermis (E) from the face of a pale-skinned young White man. There are more melanosomes (blue) in the basal keratinocytes than in the suprabasal cells. The melanocytes (M) appear to contain very few melanosomes. The keratinocytes in the malpighian layer have a sparse concentration of melanosomes (red). In spite of a sparse distribution of melanosomes in the epidermis, there are a few melanophages in the dermis (D) which have ingested melanosomes (green). OM 400x. Courtesy of Dr. W. H. Fahrenbach.

B. Epidermis (E) from the face of a young Black woman. There are numerous melanosomes (red) everywhere in the malpighian layer and in the basal layer (blue); the melanosomes are very densely packed. Note the pendulous melanocytes (P). In the papillary dermis (D) are many melanosomes (green) inside the melanophages. Generally, the abundance of melanosomes in the dermis is directly related to the darkness of the skin. OM 400x. Courtesy of Dr. W. H. Fahrenbach.

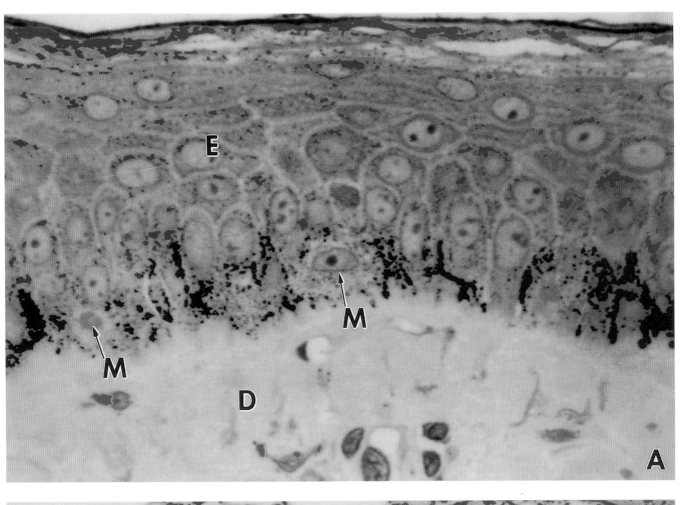

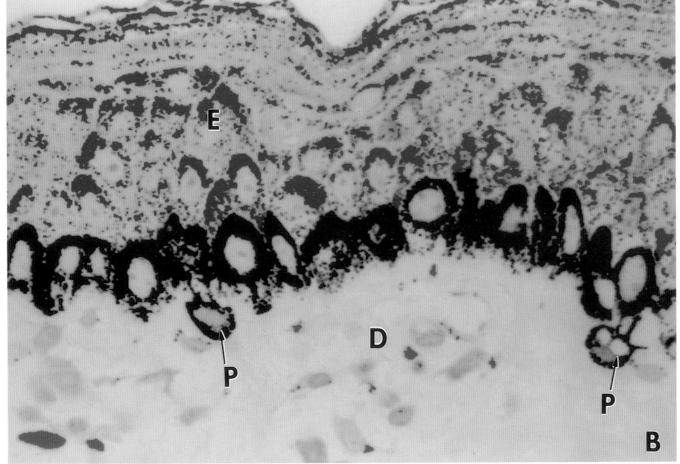

PLATE 29

KERATINOCYTES

Melanosomes

The packaging of the melanosomes within keratinocytes depends on the size of the melanosome. The large melanosomes in Black skin are single and, as a rule, individually membrane-bound. The smaller melanosomes in White skin are aggregated in complexes enclosed by a membrane.

A. In this TEM micrograph of keratinocytes in White skin epidermis, the melanosomes are small and roundish (about 0.5 μm in diameter), and relatively sparse. Nuclei (N). OM 4500x. Courtesy of Dr. G. Szabo and E. Flynn.

B. Melanosome complexes inside keratinocytes of White skin. In White skin, the pigment granules are of variable size and shape and are clustered within membrane-bound packages. OM 13,000x.

C. Numerous individual elliptical melanosomes that average about 1 μm in length are in the basal layer of Black skin keratinocytes. Nuclei (N). OM 4500x. Courtesy of Dr. G. Szabo and E. Flynn.

D. The melanosomes in Black skin remain mostly as single entities, each enclosed within a membrane (arrows). OM 13,000x.

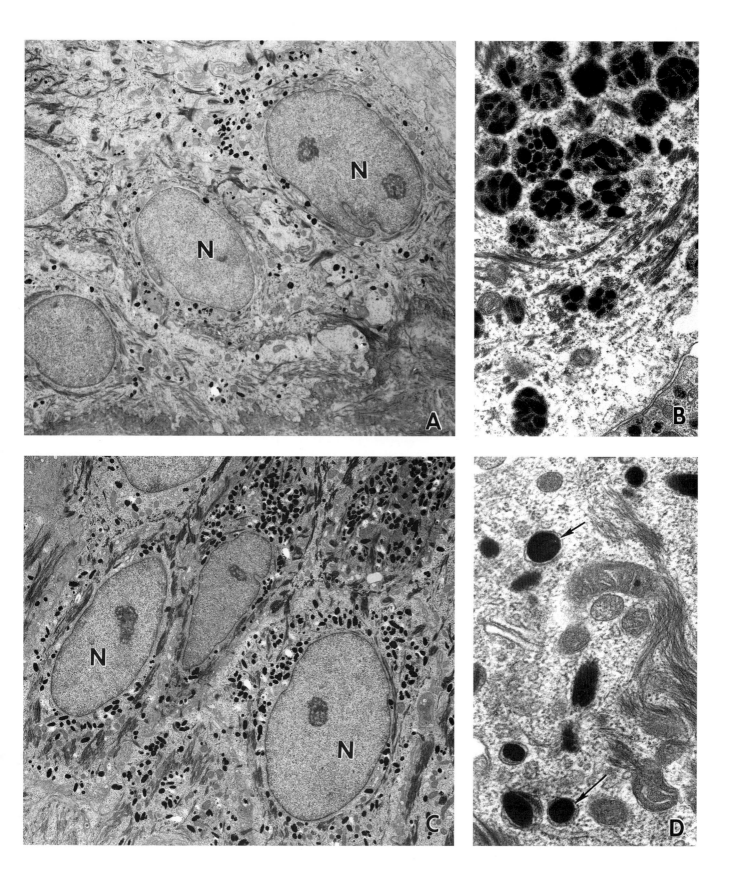

PLATE 30

DENDRITIC CELLS

Melanocytes and Langerhans Cells

Melanocytes and Langerhans cells are the only dendritic cells of the epidermis. They have no tonofibrils and do not form desmosomal junctions with adjacent cells. The best way to demonstrate epidermal melanocytes is in a split-skin epidermal sheath treated with the dopa reaction (3,4-dihydroxyphenylalanine). A positive dopa reaction indicates active tyrosinase, an enzyme of the biosynthetic pathway to melanin (converts tyrosine to melanin). Langerhans cells have no positive dopa reaction, but they can be demonstrated histochemically by staining for adenosine triphosphatase (ATPase).

A. Dopa-reactive melanocytes in an epidermal split-skin sheath of the festooned inferior border of the lower eyelid of a young White man. The only "stain" used here is dopa, for the histochemical demonstration of tyrosinase. Dopa technique. OM 400x.

B. These dendritic cells are Langerhans cells from a razor-shave biopsy specimen that was treated for the presence of ATPase. Langerhans cells are said to make up only 5% of the population of normal epidermis. OM 100x.

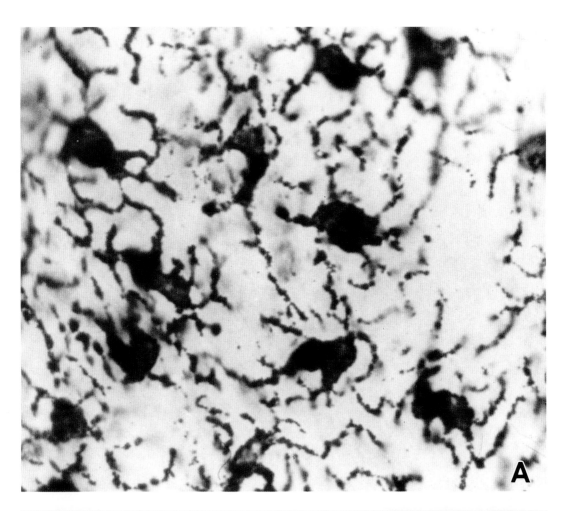

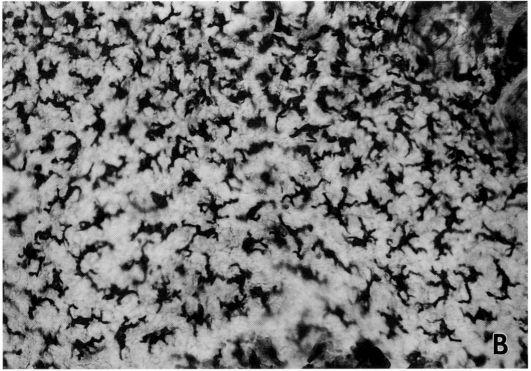

PLATE 31

LANGERHANS CELL

A. TEM micrograph of an epidermal Langerhans cell with an indented nucleus (N). This cell is unequivocally identified at the ultrastructural level by the laminated organelles, the Birbeck granules (G), in the cytoplasm. There are no keratin filaments in the cytoplasm or desmosomes on the cell membrane. Langerhans cells are antigen-presenting cells of the peripheral immune system. Mitochondrion (M). OM 15,000x. Inset: Enlarged tennis racket-shaped Birbeck granules. OM 80,000x. Courtesy of Dr. F. Hu.

B. Cytoplasm of another Langerhans cell showing many Birbeck granules (G) and mitochondria (M) scattered in the cell. Langerhans cells also contain ribosomes, lysosomes, endoplasmic reticulum, and Golgi complexes. OM 30,000x. Inset: The trilaminar structure of the Birbeck granules is clearly seen. OM 100,000x. Courtesy of Dr. Mary Bell.

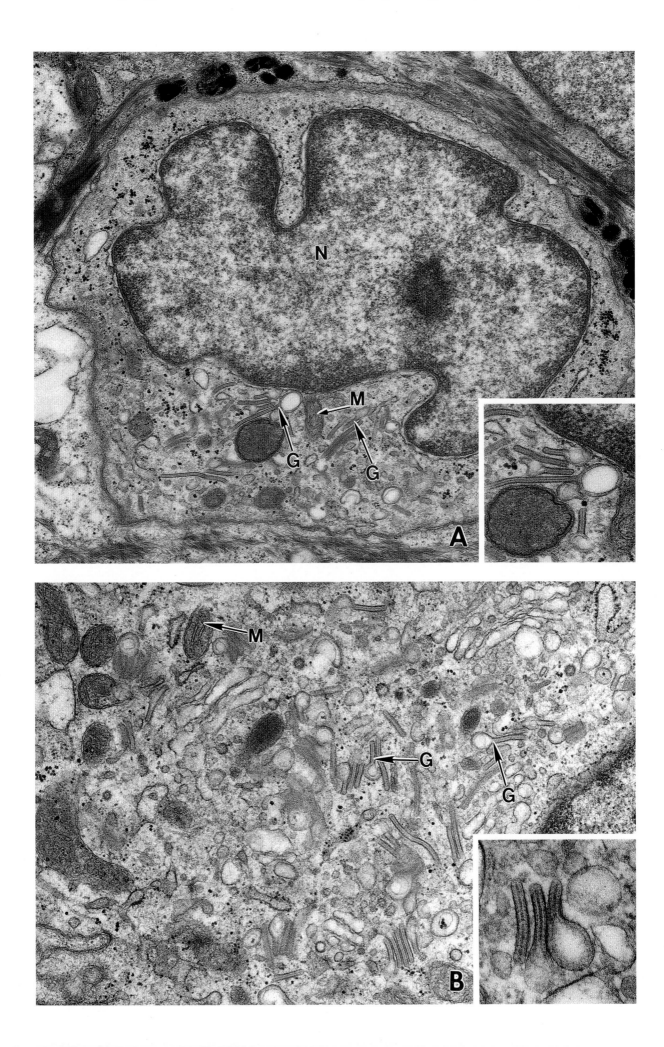

PLATE 32

IMMUNOCYTOCHEMISTRY LANGERHANS CELL

Laser scanning confocal microscopy is a new and powerful cyto-chemical technique. This epidermis has been immunocytochemical-ly labeled for neural cell adhesion molecule to define unmyelinated dermal axons (bright red), and for CD1 to define epidermal Langer-hans cells and their dendrites (yellow-green). The blue background region is the keratinocytes. This image is a computer-assisted sum-mation of seven "optical" sections, each obtained at 2-μm intervals. This technique facilitates an appreciation of the complex spatial associations among skin cells. This section suggests a connection between Langerhans cells and intraepidermal axons. Courtesy of Dr. George Murphy.

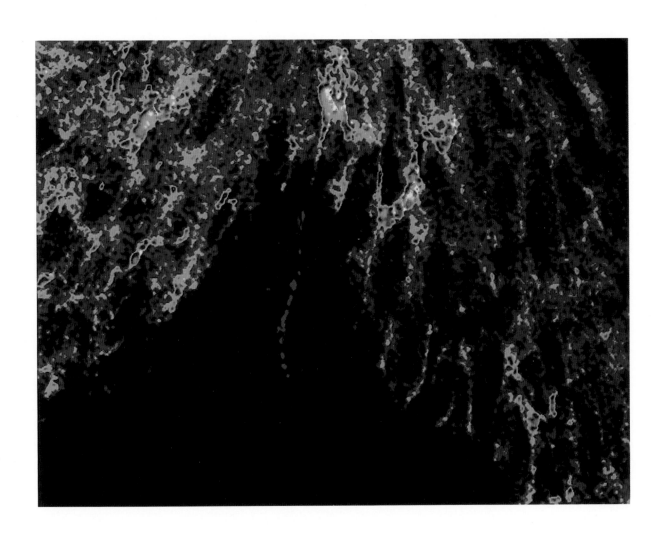

PLATE 33

MERKEL CELL

Merkel cells, located in the basal part of the epidermis, are characterized by membrane-bound, dense-core granules. There is evidence that Merkel cells are associated with intraepidermal neurites (act as transducers). The Merkel cell is believed to be a type I mechanoreceptor. The function of these cells, however, is not definitely known.

A. TEM micrograph of the cytoplasm of a Merkel cell (M) containing many dense secretory granules (arrows). Desmosomes (D) join these cells to the keratinocytes (K). From the back of the hand of a 65-year-old man. OM 9000x.

B. TEM micrograph of a Merkel cell (M) near a healing wound, with characteristic dense granules (arrows); two axons (A) accompany the cell. There are keratinocytes around the Merkel cell. Basal lamina (BL). OM 6000x. Courtesy of Dr. B. Munger and Dr. L. Dellon.

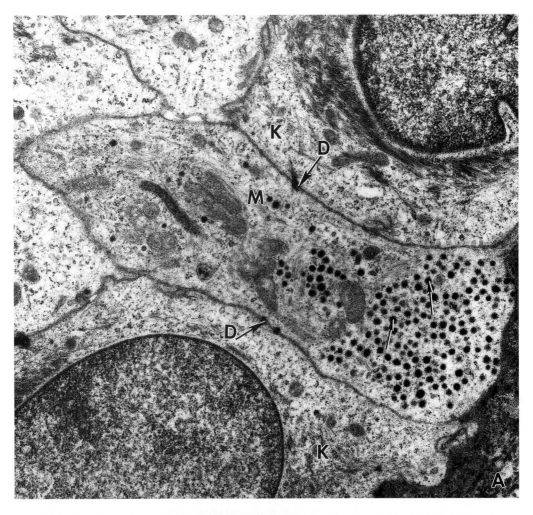

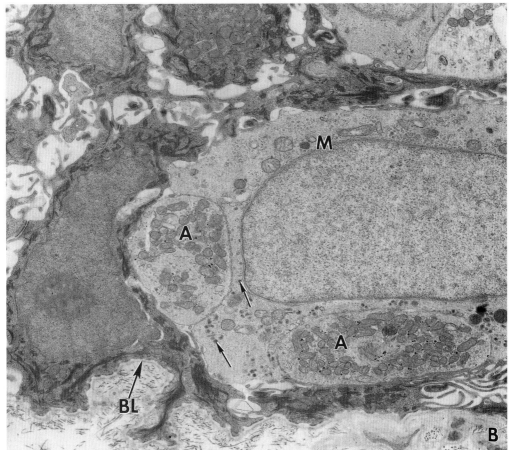

PLATE 34

MICRORADIOGRAPHY of EPIDERMIS

A unique approach to the study of skin histology is that of microradiography using ultrasoft x-rays; the degree of absorption of the x-rays is dependent on dry mass. Another approach is to irradiate the specimen with ultraviolet light and look at the photoabsorption.

A. This paraffin-embedded section of normal skin shows the different amounts of absorption (due to differences in dry mass concentration of proteins) following microradiography using ultrasoft x-rays in the epidermal malpighian layer and stratum corneum, and in the papillary and reticular dermis. OM 100x. Courtesy of Prof. Antonio Tosti.

B. Higher magnification of the spinous-layer keratinocytes of an unstained epidermis in a paraffin section exposed to ultrasoft x-rays (0.7 kV). The cytoplasm (C) and nucleoli (No), which appear white, show greater x-ray absorption than the nuclei (N). OM 630x. Courtesy of Prof. Antonio Tosti.

C. This contact photomicrograph of an unstained paraffin section exposed to ultraviolet light (2580 nm) shows the pronounced ultraviolet photoabsorption of melanin (arrows) in the basal cells and of the nucleic acids in all epidermal cells. OM 250x. Courtesy of Prof. Antonio Tosti.

D. The same section of skin as in Figure C, stained with H and E, shows a heavily melanized epidermis in a dark-skinned person. OM 250x. Courtesy of Prof. Antonio Tosti.

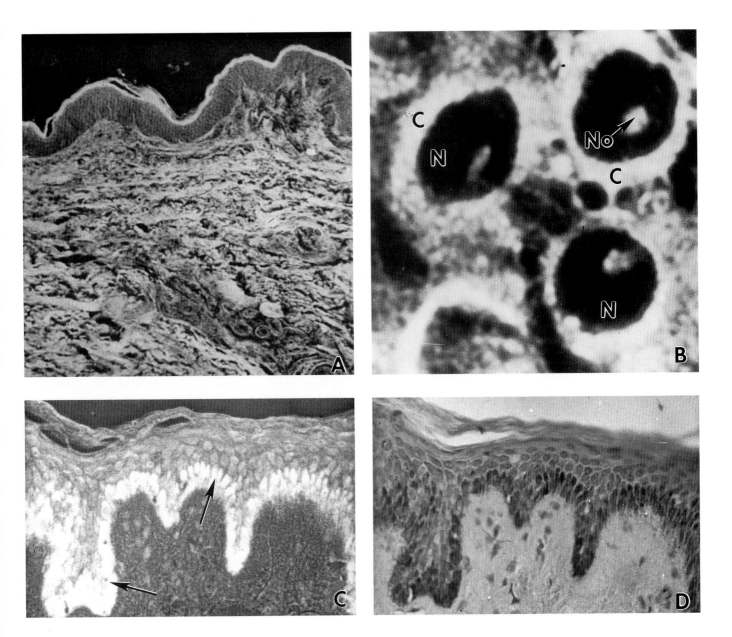

PLATE 35

EPIDERMIS PHOTODAMAGE

Photodamage is the gross and microscopic changes that occur in the skin as a result of solar radiation. It is likely that damage in the epidermis reflects relatively recent solar exposure, since the differentiation of a basal cell requires about 28 days.

A. Exposure to the sun has damaged this epidermis in the facial skin of a young White woman. Many of the keratinocytes (arrow) and melanocytes (M) are vacuolated. Atypia, atrophy, necrosis, and abnormal staining patterns are seen in the keratinocytes. Under the epidermis is the Grenz zone (Gr), free of the normal oxytalan and elaunin fibers. 2-μm plastic section. H and Lee. OM 630x. Reproduced with permission of Richardson-Vicks, a Procter and Gamble Company, from Montagna, Carlisle and Kirchner, *Epidermal and Dermal Histological Markers of Photodamaged Human Facial Skin*. 1989.

B. This grossly sun-damaged epidermis from the face of a young woman has a swollen stratum lucidum (L) with vesicles (V) full of stainable material. There are vacuolated and atypic keratinocytes throughout the epidermis. Stratum granulosum (G). Elastic fibers (E). Grenz zone (Gr). 2-μm plastic section. H and Lee. OM 400x. Used with permission of Richardson-Vicks, a Procter and Gamble Company. From Montagna, Carlisle and Kirchner, *Epidermal and Dermal Histological Markers of Photodamaged Human Facial Skin*. 1989.

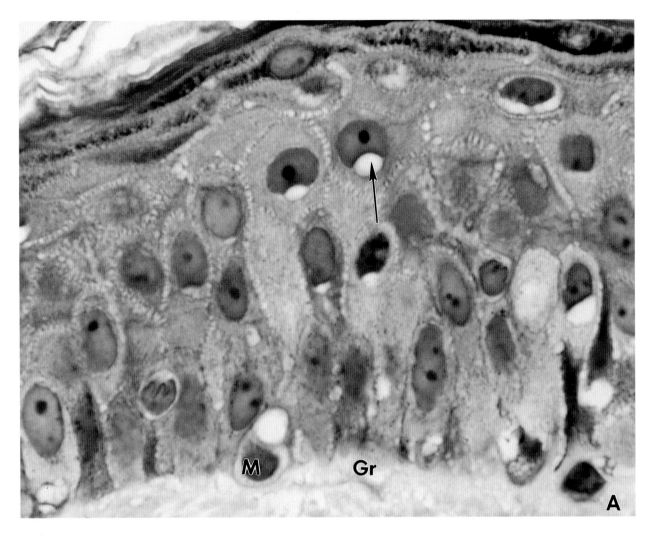

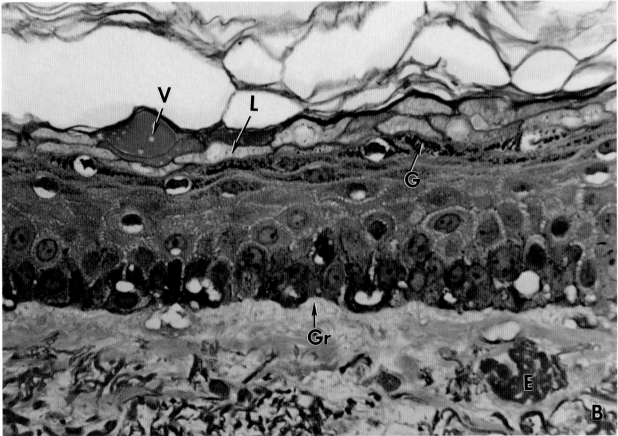

PLATE 36

EPIDERMIS PHOTODAMAGE

Excessive sun exposure causes drastic changes in the keratinocytes. In addition, the melanocytes become large, more branched, and produce more melanosomes; they are often vacuolated. There is a decrease in the number of functional Langerhans cells.

A. This sun-damaged epidermis from the face of a young woman shows severe degenerative changes. Many keratinocytes are necrotic, vacuolated, and vary in size, shape, and staining properties (atypia). The stratum lucidum (L) is thick and swollen, with vesicles (V) full of materials that stain differently from the cytoplasm of the other stratum lucidum cells. Intercellular edema is evident. 2-μm plastic section. H and Lee. OM 630x.

B. Keratohyalin granules (K) in the granular layer stain red with picrosirius red in the sun-damaged facial skin epidermis of a young White woman. The cells of the stratum lucidum (L), also stained red, are swollen. The material inside the vesicles (V), typical of severe photodamage, remains unstained. 2-μm plastic section. OM 630x.

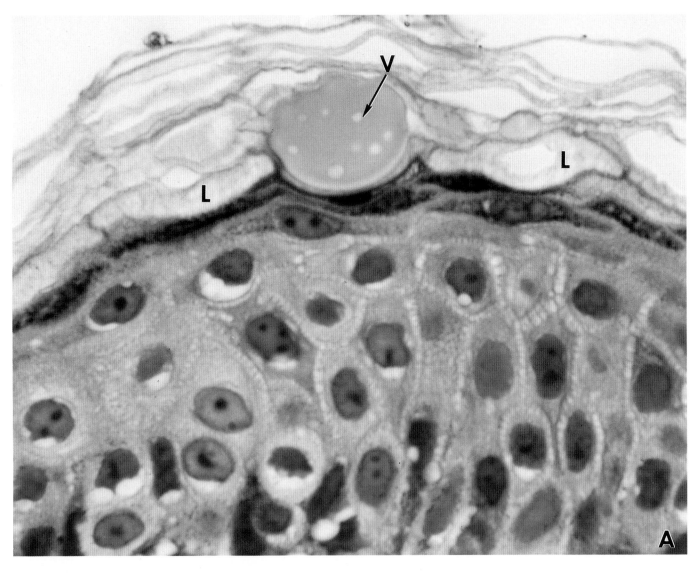

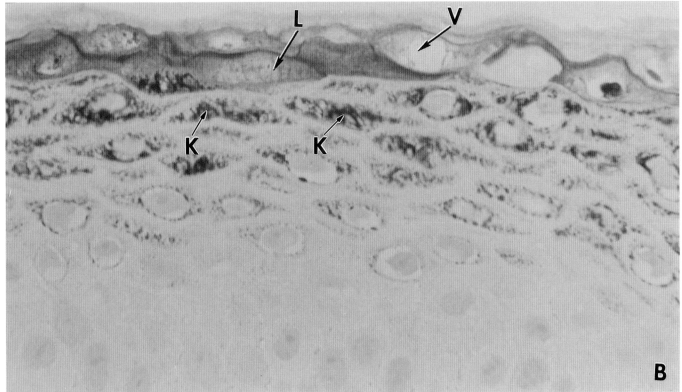

PLATE 37

SOLAR LENTIGINES

Solar lentigines, also known as liver spots, are benign lesions that have a tendency to occur on photodamaged skin. In middle age, scarcely a White person is spared the development of solar lentigines on the sun-exposed hands, wrists, arms, neck, and face. The hyperpigmented, flat spots are a result of hyperplastic melanocytes that produce great quantities of pigment. This is a TEM micrograph of vacuolated (V) basal keratinocytes from a solar lentigo from the wrist of a 65-year-old man. Note the dense accumulation of various-sized aggregated melanosome complexes (arrows). Nucleus (N). Nucleolus (No). Papillary dermis (PD). Basal lamina (BL). OM 5000x.

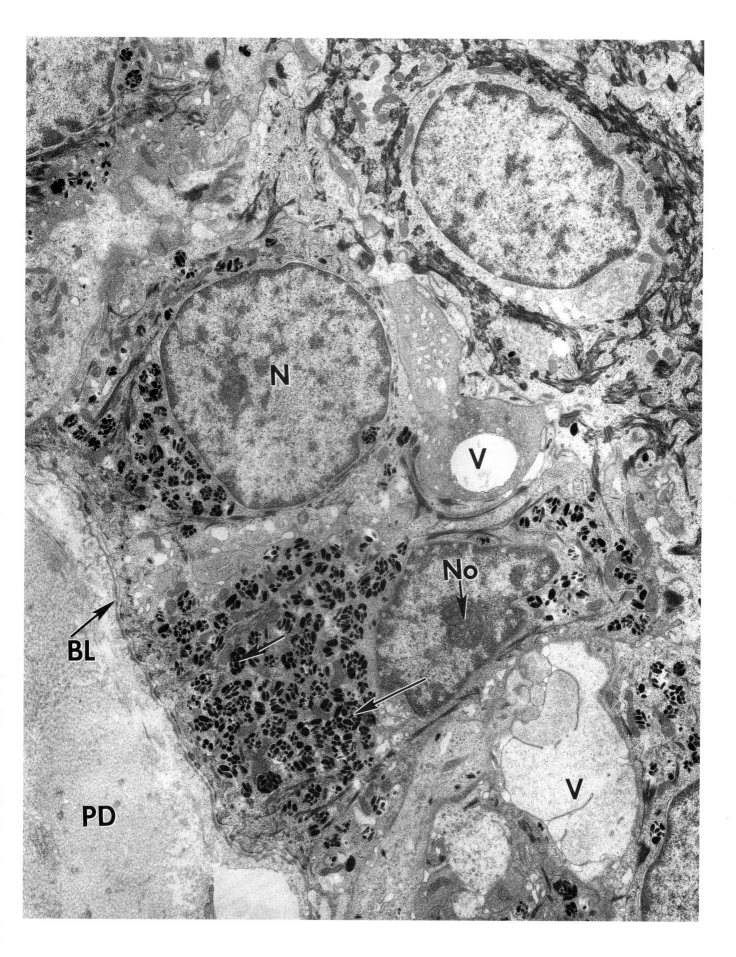

PLATE 38

EPIDERMIS
Aging

A. This epidermis from the cheek skin of a dark-skinned 73-year-old White man shows mild sun damage. There are some intercellular edema and a few vacuoles in keratinocytes and melanocytes (M). Note the blunted, thick cytoplasmic processes (arrows) that remain on the basal keratinocytes in spite of age and photodamage. 2-μm plastic section. H and Lee. OM 1000x.

B. In this trunk skin epidermis from the same 73-year-old man, the keratinocytes are variable in size, shape, and staining properties. The abnormal columnar basal cells have a dense cytoplasm and are referred to as "dark" cells (D). There is considerable vacuolization, even though this skin had not been directly exposed to the sun for at least 4 years. A dilated subepidermal blood vessel (BV) is typical of older skin. 2-μm plastic section. H and Lee. OM 630x.

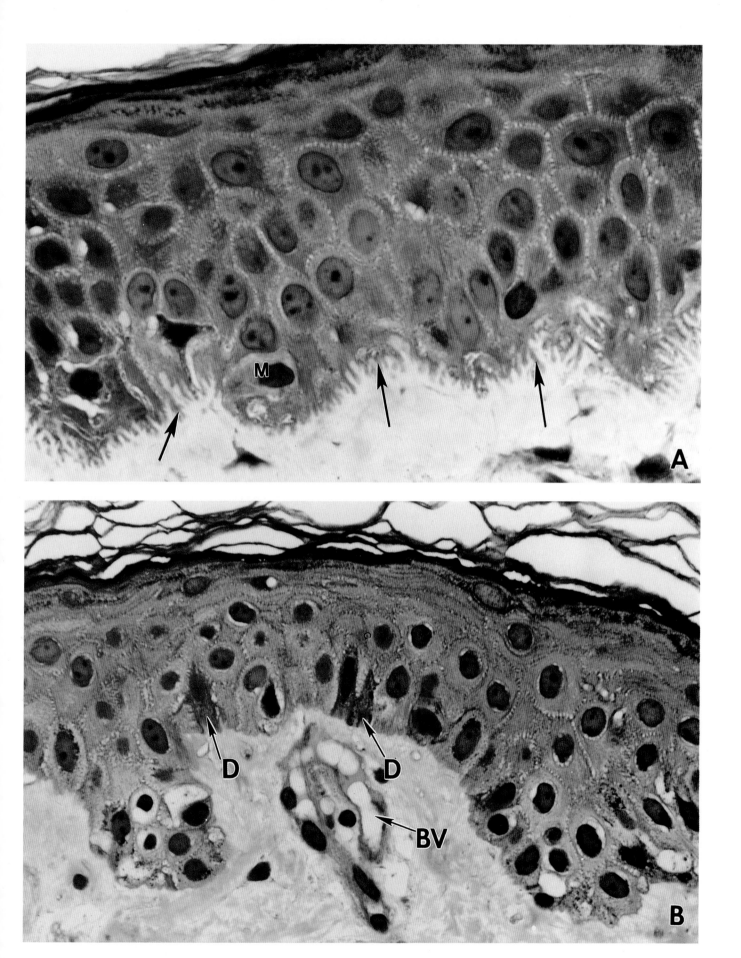

PLATE 39

UNDERSIDE of EPIDERMIS

A. SEM micrograph of skin that was immersed in a sodium bromide solution, then the epidermis (Ep) was peeled from the dermis (De). The dermal projections fit into the corresponding epidermal depressions. The ducts (Dt) of two eccrine sweat glands remain attached to the epidermis, and two hair follicles (arrow) are on the dermal side. OM 25x.

B. SEM micrograph of the underside of split palmar epidermis showing alternating ridges and valleys. The papillary dermis mirrors the contours of the epidermis. The papillae of the dermis fit into the holes along the ridges of the epidermal underside. OM 80x. Courtesy of Dr. W. H. Fahrenbach.

C. Higher magnification shows that the entire underside of the epidermis is covered with fine cytoplasmic rootlets that extend from the basal keratinocytes and give the epidermal underside a velvet-like appearance. Note the duct of a sweat gland (DSG). OM 500x. Courtesy of Dr. W. H. Fahrenbach.

D. The basal extensions are clearly seen in this highly magnified SEM micrograph of keratinocytes. These extensions are better developed in the skin of the friction surfaces and the elbows, knees, and face than they are in the skin of other parts of the body. OM 2000x. Courtesy of Dr. W. H. Fahrenbach.

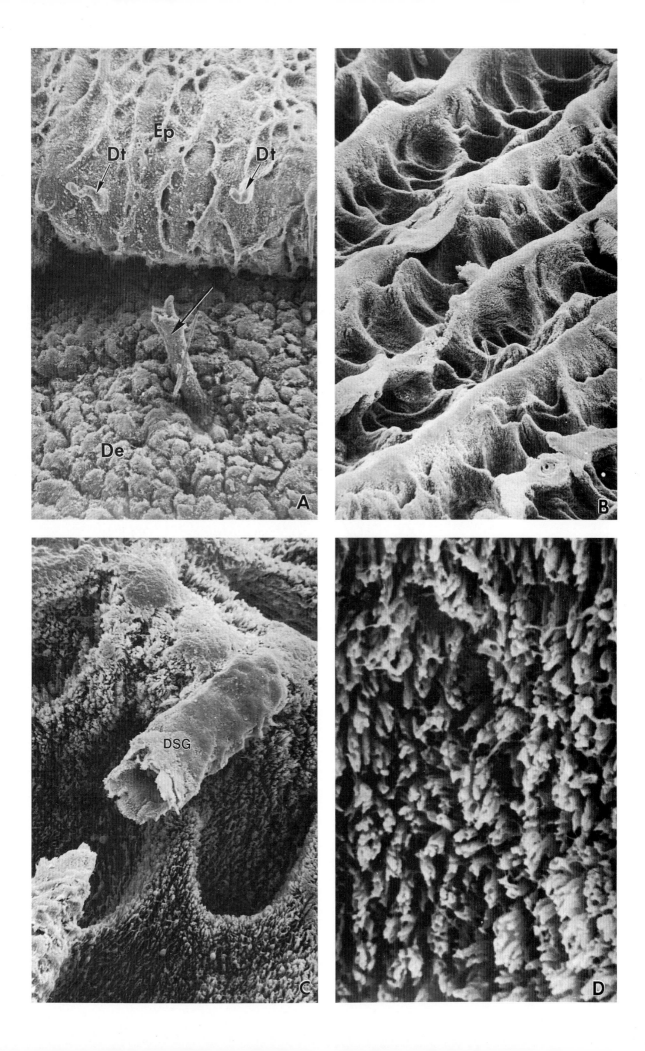

PLATE 40

UNDERSIDE of EPIDERMIS

Visualization of the undersurface of the epidermis after the skin has been immersed in sodium bromide shows a complex architecture and uneven terrain. The split-skin preparations show great regional variations similar to the variations seen in histological sections of the dermal–epidermal junctions.

A. The underside of the epidermis of the palpebral border is carunculated. The follicles of the cilia (eyelashes) (C) are surrounded by epidermal moats (arrows). OM 100x.

B. The underside of the glabrous epidermis that covers the labia minora is sculptured in swirling, leaf-like designs. The white structures (arrows) are sebaceous glands. OM 120x.

C. The underside of the epidermis of the glabrous glans penis (G) is simple and has no characteristic pattern. OM 120x.

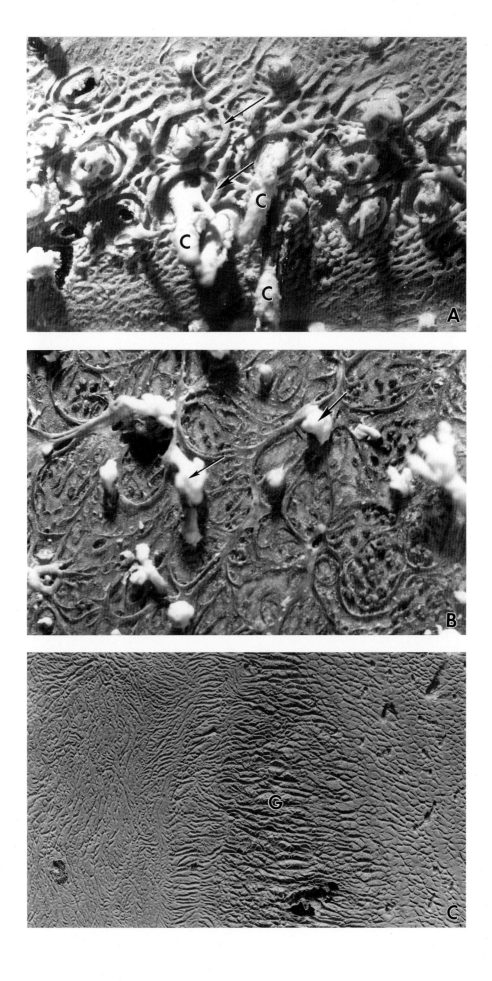

PLATE 41

UNDERSIDE of EPIDERMIS
Aging

A. The sculptured underside of the abdominal epidermis of a 17-year-old woman. The various-sized holes (arrows) were occupied by the papillary dermis. Such an architecture provides a greater interface between the epidermis and the dermis. Split-skin preparation. OM 100x.

B. During the aging process, the epidermis becomes thinner and the dermal–epidermal junction flattens, as in this epidermis of the abdominal skin of a 92-year-old woman. There are fewer and more distorted "holes," and the ridges are considerably lower, thinner, and farther apart than in younger epidermis. Split-skin preparation. OM 100x.

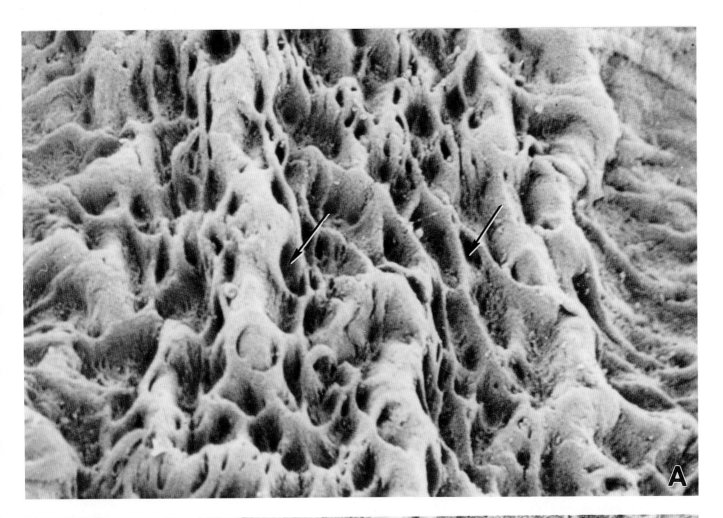

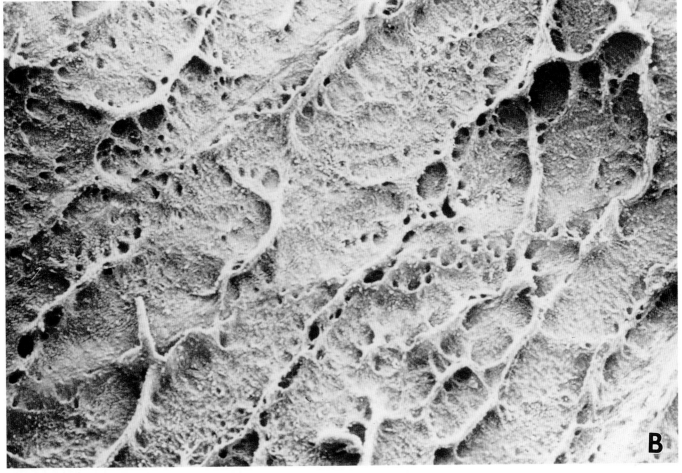

PLATE 42

BASEMENT MEMBRANE

At the dermal–epidermal junction, a PAS-reactive basement membrane follows the contour of the basal cells. The basement membrane physically and functionally separates the epidermis from the dermis.

A. Epidermis from the malar eminence of a 35-year-old White woman. The crinkly basement membrane (BM) is strongly PAS-reactive. 4-μm plastic section. PAS counterstained with hematoxylin. OM 630x.

B. The PAS-reactive basement membrane (BM) of the thick epidermis in the volar surface of the finger of a 36-year-old man. The cytoplasmic extensions in the basal cells are more prominent than in thin epidermis. 4-μm plastic section. PAS counterstained with hematoxylin. OM 1000x.

C. Epidermis from the malar eminence of a young woman. The reticulin fibers (RF) that accompany the basement membrane appear like a row of commas; reticulin is believed to be newly synthesized type I or III collagen. 2-μm plastic section. Gridley's reticulin fiber technique. OM 630x.

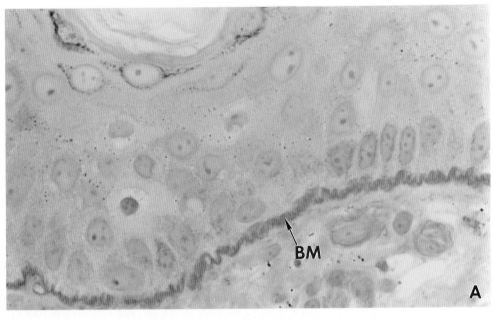

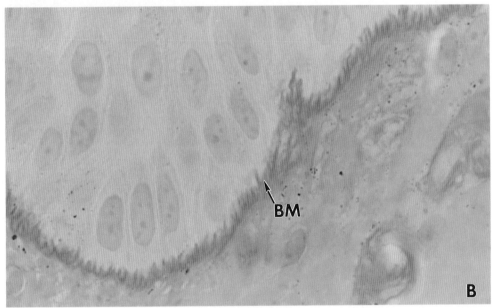

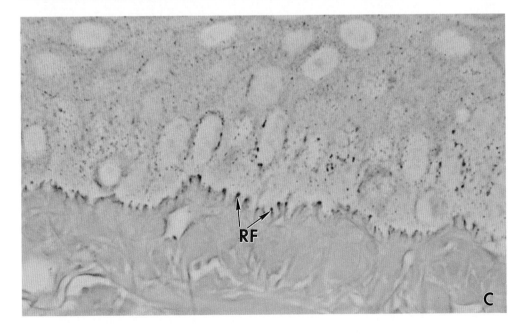

PLATE 43

DERMAL–EPIDERMAL JUNCTION

TEM micrograph of the dermal–epidermal junction. The basal lamina, which is both a boundary and an interface, provides a functional and structural separation between the epidermis and the papillary dermis. Interactions occur between the two layers that are dependent on each other for regulation and modulation of their normal structure and function. Spinous cells, basal keratinocytes (BK), and melanocytes (M) are seen in the epidermis. Various dermal cells are scattered among the collagen bundles (C) in the papillary dermis. Nerve endings (N) surrounded by Schwann cells are directly below the epidermis. 3500x. Courtesy of Douglas R. Keene.

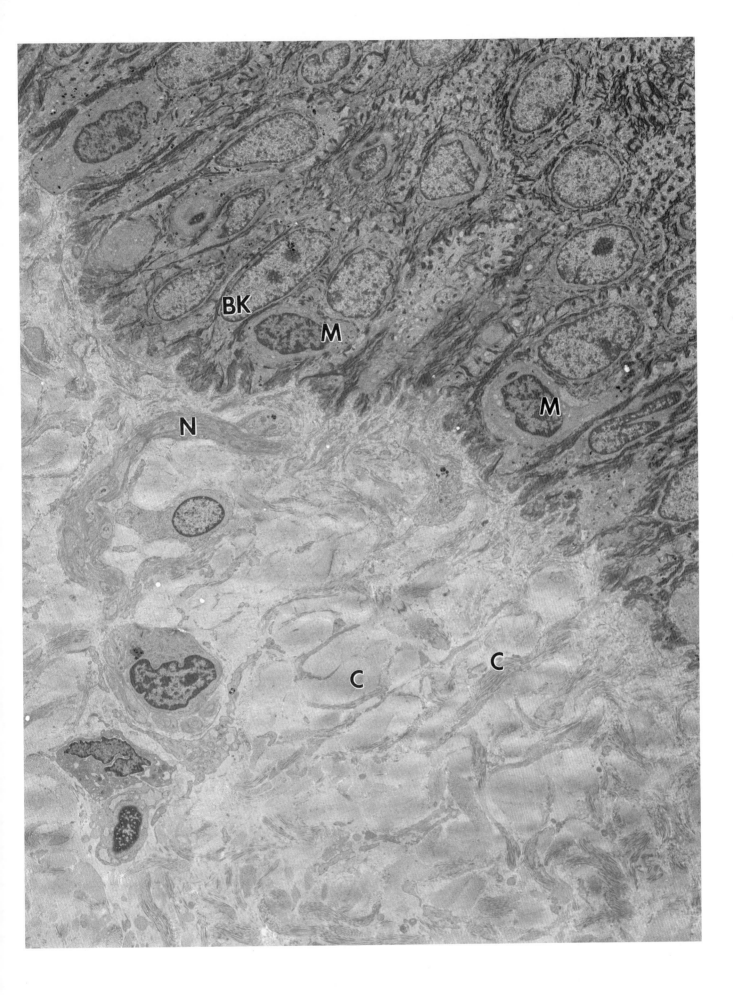

PLATE 44

BASEMENT MEMBRANE

A. TEM micrograph of the basal lamina between the epidermis and the papillary dermis (PD). The basal lamina functions as a structural foundation for the epidermal basal cells, a barrier between the epidermis and the dermis, and an attachment site for the dermis to the epidermis. Basal keratinocytes (K) produce the hemidesmosomes (hd), anchoring filaments (af), lamina lucida (LL), and lamina densa (LD). The anchoring fibrils (AF) are synthesized by the dermal fibroblasts. The hemidesmosome is a junction between the basal keratinocyte and the lamina densa; keratin filaments (kf) attach to the specialized junction within the keratinocyte, and anchoring filaments attach to the dermal side. The lamina lucida contains glycoproteins that are important for adhesion between the epidermal cells and the lamina densa. The lamina densa acts as a filter and a structural scaffold for the attachment of the epidermal basal cells at one surface, and the elastin–collagen matrix on the dermal side. The anchoring fibrils are short, banded fibrils that originate at the lamina densa. OM 20,000x.

B. The basal lamina (BL) provides a series of attachments of the dermal components with the epidermal basal cells. Anchoring fibrils (AF), which are collagenous components, connect the dermal collagen (C) directly with the lamina densa. The elastic network inserts into the basal lamina by way of the elastic microfibrils (El), the oxytalan fibers. Keratin filaments (kf) form a cytoskeleton within the keratinocyte (K) and attach to a hemidesmosome (hd). Papillary dermis (PD). OM 14,000x.

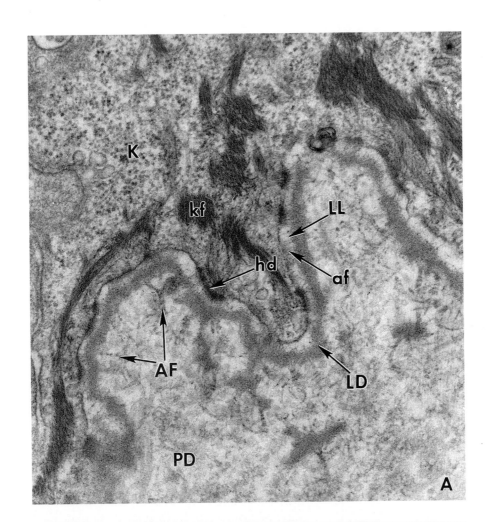

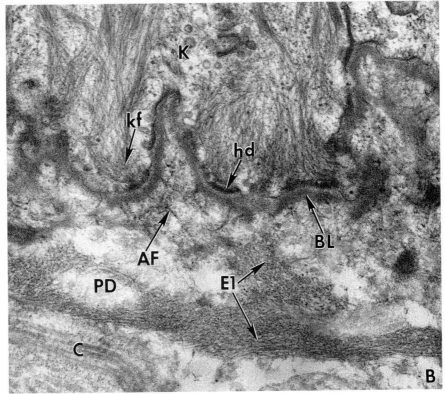

PLATE 45

BASEMENT MEMBRANE

Type VII Collagen, Kalinin

EM immunolocalization of type VII collagen and the protein, kalinin, in the dermal–epidermal junction of human neonatal foreskin.

A. The adherence of the basal keratinocytes to the dermis is mediated by hemidesmosomes (hd), electron-dense thickenings along the plasma membrane of basal cells. The hemidesmosomes contain transmembrane proteins that interact with the keratin filaments (kf) on the cytoplasmic side, and with anchoring filaments (af) that traverse the lamina lucida (ll) of the basal lamina and insert into the lamina densa (ld). Anchoring fibrils (AFi) appear to originate in the lamina densa, extend into the papillary dermis, encircle the banded collagen fibers, and reinsert back into the lamina densa. Anchoring fibrils originating in the lamina densa also extend into the dermis where they insert into electron-dense anchoring plaques (AP). Additional anchoring fibrils span these plaques, forming a network that entraps many dermal fibrous elements and secures the lamina densa to the dermis. Monoclonal antibodies specific for type VII collagen and gold-conjugated secondary antibodies are found at the ends of anchoring fibrils,within the lamina densa of the basal lamina and the anchoring plaques. Type VII collagen is the only known component of the anchoring fibrils. OM 67,000x. Courtesy of Robert E. Burgeson and Douglas R. Keene.

B. Diagram of the basement membrane zone; the types of collagens known to exist in the various components are indicated. Courtesy of Robert E. Burgeson and Douglas R. Keene. Reproduced from the *Journal of Cell Biology*, 1987, 104: 620 by copyright permission of the Rockefeller University Press.

C. Antibodies specific to the protein kalinin and silver-amplified, colloidal gold-conjugated secondary antibodies localize to the anchoring filaments (arrows). OM 50,400x. Courtesy of Robert E. Burgeson and Douglas R. Keene.

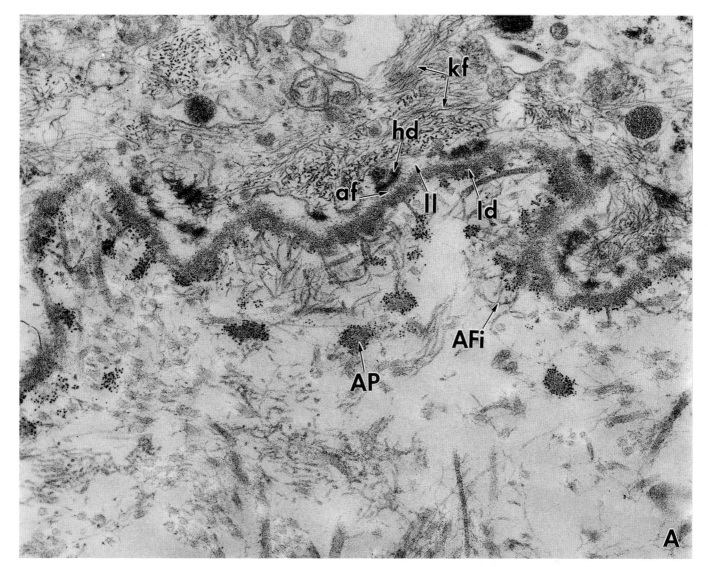

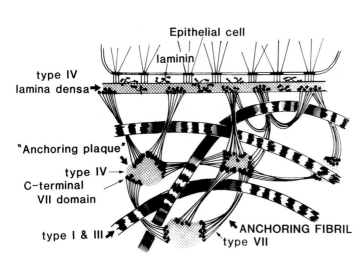

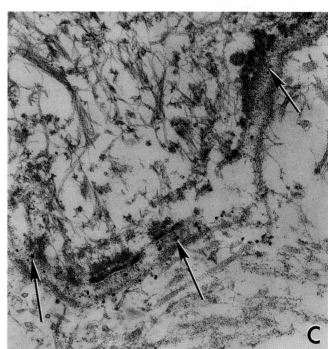

Dermis

The dermis, the connective tissue matrix of the skin, makes up 15 to 20% of the total body weight. It gives the skin its structural strength, protects the body from injury, stores water, and interacts with the epidermis. Nerves, vascular networks, and skin appendages are supported in the dermal extracellular matrix, which consists of collagen and elastic fibers, filamentous structures, and an amorphous ground substance. The recognition of the cells in the dermis has always been a challenge to histologists, but the electron microscope has resolved this problem. Fibroblasts, macrophages, mast cells, and lymphocytes are the resident cells of the dermis.

PLATE 46

FIBROBLASTS

Fibroblasts are more numerous in the papillary dermis than in the reticular dermis. They give rise to fibers and the ground substance of the extracellular matrix; in addition, they can remove the fibers by secreting enzymes such as collagenase and elastase. Fibroblasts also synthesize some parts of the basement membrane. Fibroblasts are the "master" cells of the dermis.

A. Fibroblasts are not only more numerous but also usually larger in the papillary dermis than in the reticular dermis. This fibroblast (F) is from the papillary layer of the facial skin of a 21-year-old Black woman. 2-μm plastic section. H and Lee. OM 800x.

B. Binucleated or multinucleated fibroblasts (arrows) are more often present in the dermis of Black facial skin than in White skin. From the same section as Figure A. H and Lee. OM 250x.

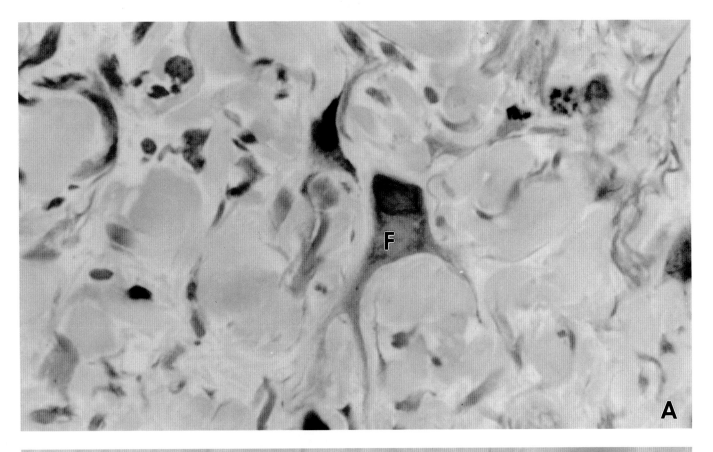

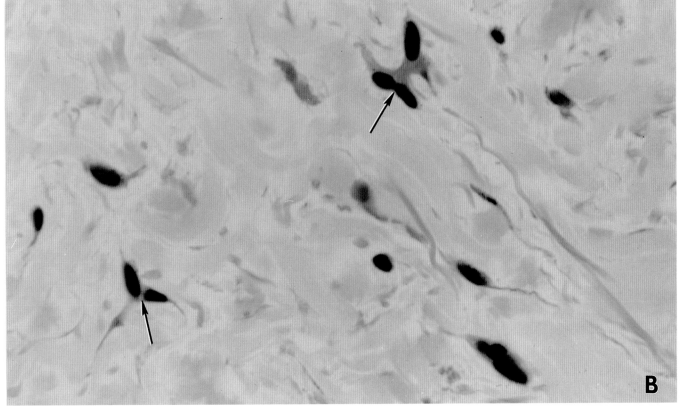

PLATE 47

PAPILLARY DERMIS

A. TEM micrograph of a fibroblast in the papillary dermis of the facial skin of a young Black woman. The plasma membrane of the fibroblast is close to the basal lamina (BL), directly below the epidermal keratinocytes (K). The dermis nourishes and influences epidermal structure and function. The cytoplasm of the fibroblast is filled with organelles including abundant rough endoplasmic reticulum (RER) and mitochondria (M). The nucleus (N) contains dispersed chromatin and a nucleolus. Collagen (C) surrounds the fibroblast. OM 6800x.

B. Portion of a fibroblast in the papillary dermis of the face of a young White woman. Fibroblasts in the papillary dermis have greater synthetic capabilities than those in the reticular dermis. The numerous organelles in this cell reflect the high metabolic activity; note the Golgi complexes (G), ribosomes and rough endoplasmic reticulum (RER), vesicles, filaments, mitochondria (M), and nucleus (N). Free nerve endings (Ne) are located in the papillary dermis below the keratinocytes (K) and the basal lamina (BL). OM 6800x.

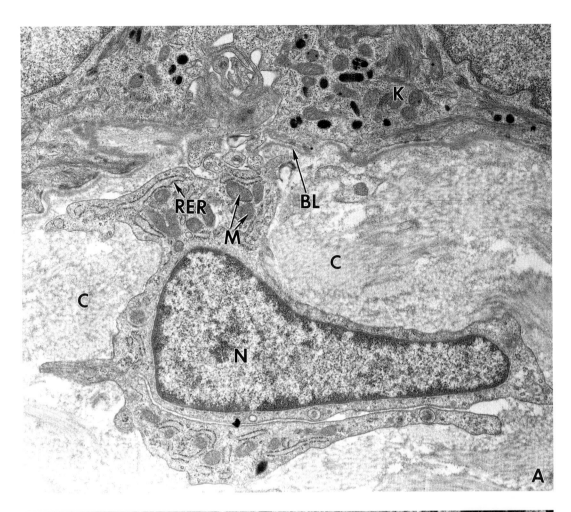

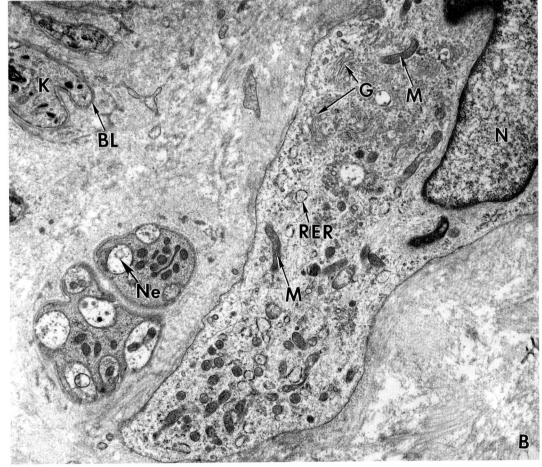

PLATE 48

ULTRASTRUCTURE of FIBROBLAST

The appearance of fibroblasts varies according to their activity. Cell size, and the abundance and appearance of the rough endoplasmic reticulum, Golgi complexes, vesicles and vacuoles, mitochondria, focal densities along the plasma membrane, nucleus, and nucleoli, all suggest the level of metabolic activity in the cell. This large, active-appearing fibroblast from the face of a young Black woman has two nuclei (Nu) , abundant rough endoplasmic reticulum (ER), Golgi bodies (G), vesicles, and filaments. Fibroblasts synthesize the fibrous materials, collagen (C) and elastin (E), which surround this cell. Many small, filamentous structures (arrows), perhaps synthesized by the fibroblast, are outside the cell membrane. Mitochondria (M) provide energy in the form of ATP. OM 8100x.

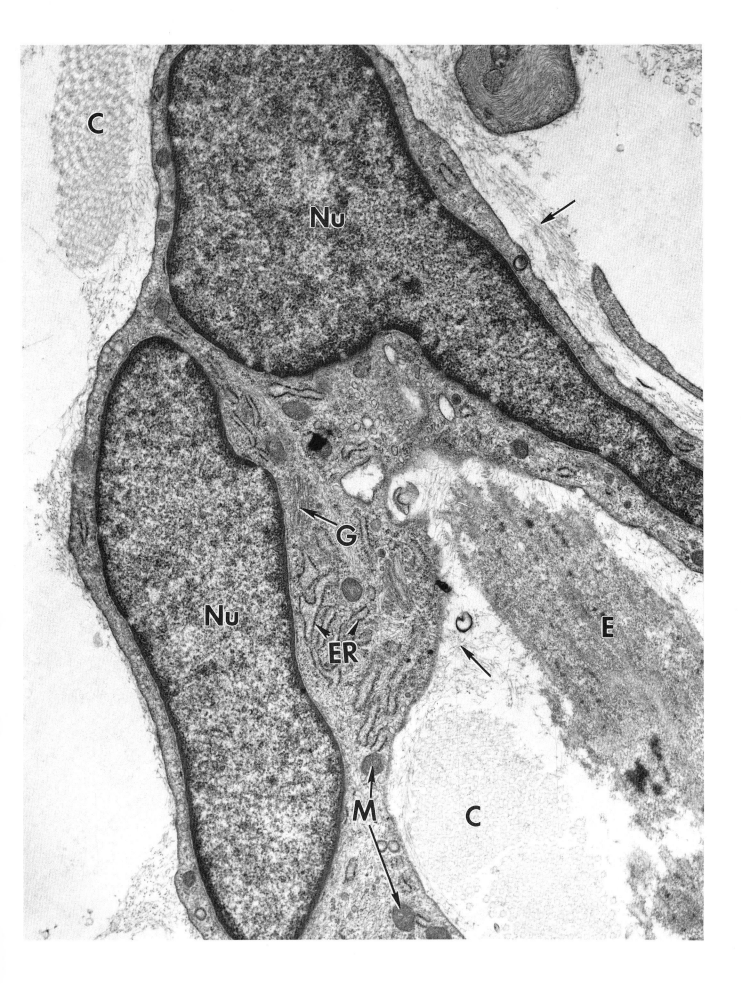

PLATE 49

FIBROBLAST

Aging

A. This fibroblast from the back of the hand of a 65-year-old man has a nucleus (N) with a prominent nucleolus (No). With advancing age, fibroblasts generally become smaller and less active, but they are often hypertrophied in photodamaged skin. The elastic fibers (E) in this figure are very dense; they are probably in a degenerative state and reflect elastosis. Compare this fibroblast and the elastic fibers with those in the previous plate. Endoplasmic reticulum (ER). Collagen (C). OM 10,000x.

B. This portion of a fibroblast from the back of the hand of a 65-year-old man contains distended rough endoplasmic reticulum (ER) indicative of high biosynthetic activity; fibroblasts in photo-damaged skin are often hypermetabolic. The dense pigment granules are lipofuchsin granules (L), also known as "old age pigment." Lipofuchsin is a marker of old age and accumulates in many different cells. The elastic fibers (E) are very dense. Collagen (C). OM 15,000x.

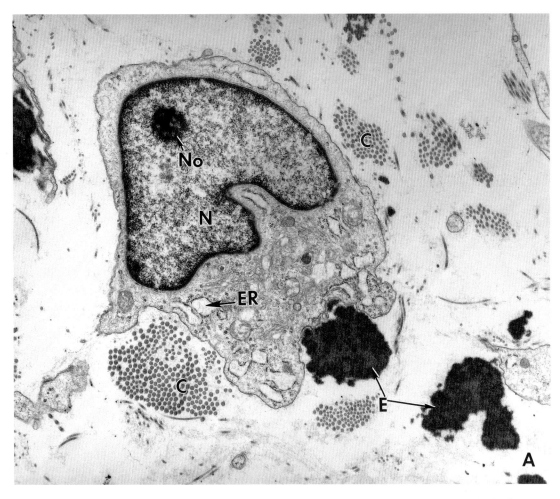

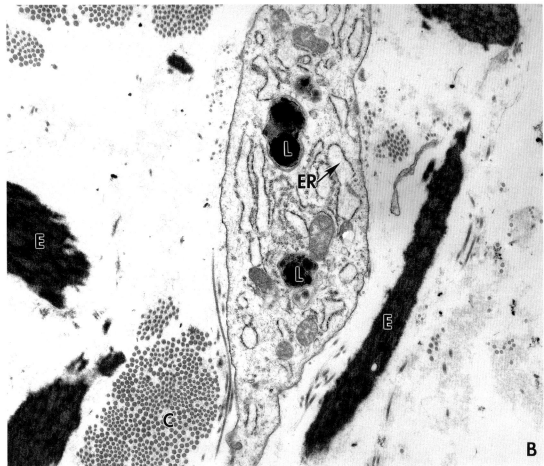

PLATE 50

FIBROBLAST

Mast Cell

The cell membrane of this fibroblast (F) abuts against the microvilli (Mi) of a mast cell (M). These two cell types are often seen close together, which may indicate cell-to-cell communication. Mast cells have been shown to influence the amount of collagen production by fibroblasts. The cytoplasm of the fibroblast contains a flagellum (fl) and the cross section of a centriole (arrow). Protein filaments (actin filaments, microtubules, and intermediate filaments) form networks that give the cell its shape and provide a basis for internal and external movements. The cytoskeleton is often organized around centrioles. Nucleus (Nu). Distended rough endoplasmic reticulum (ER). Elastin (E). Collagen (C). From the back of the hand of a 65-year-old man. OM 10,000x.

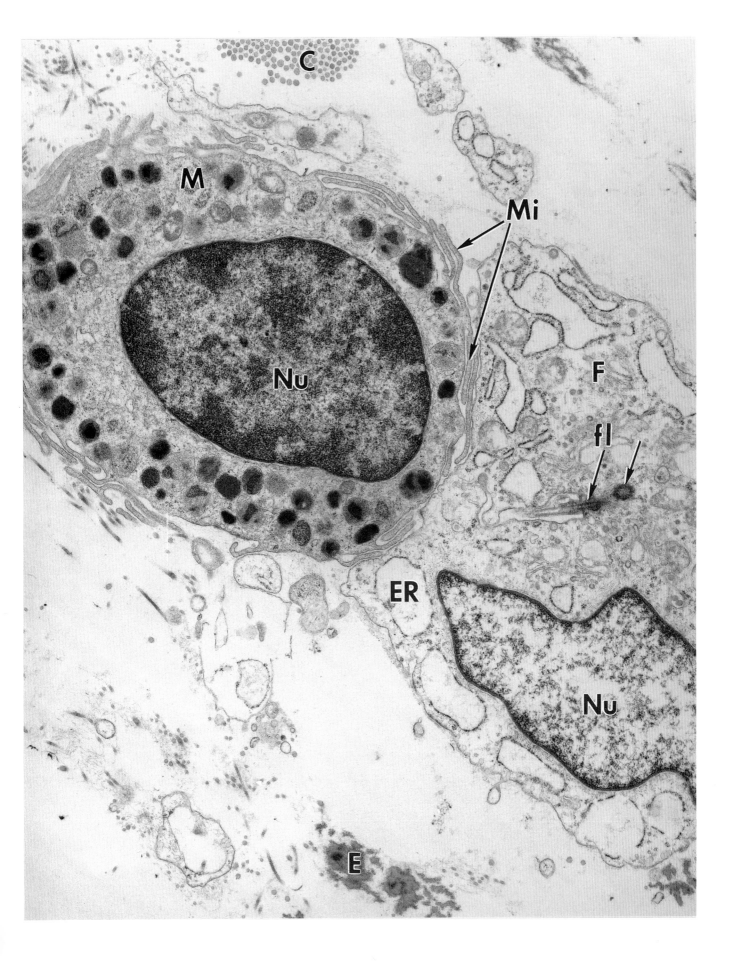

PLATE 51

MACROPHAGES

Macrophages have various structural and functional capabilities: they phagocytize cell and fiber debris, synthesize and secrete a number of hydrolytic enzymes, and participate in immune responses.

A. Phagocytic macrophages that ingest melanosomes are known as melanophages. Some melanophages are always present in the dermis, but they are also more numerous in dark skin, whether in sun-exposed or in protected areas. They are numerous in chronically inflamed skin. These cells from the face of a young Black woman contain what appear to be partially degraded melanosomes (arrows). 2-μm plastic section. H and Lee. OM 630x.

B. Large melanophage (Me) replete with melanosomes from the face of a young White woman. The smaller cell (arrow) contains ingested granules at each end of the nucleus. Mast cell (Ma). 2-μm plastic section. Giemsa stain. OM 1200x.

C. Melanophages (arrows) in the face of a young Black woman. Compare the staining of the granules in the mast cell (Ma) with the granules in the melanophages. 2-μm plastic section. Fontana-Masson silver technique counterstained with H and Lee. OM 1000x.

D. Multinucleated cell (arrow) in the papillary dermis of the face of a young Black woman, containing few melanosomes. Such cells resemble fibroblasts that have engulfed melanosomes. Melanophages filled with granules are also present; the size of the argyrophilic melanosomes and the density of their argyrophilia probably indicate the degree of the enzymatic hydrolysis. 2-μm plastic section. Fontana-Masson silver technique counterstained with nuclear fast red. OM 1000x.

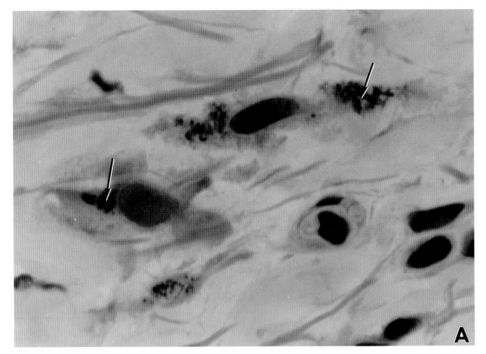
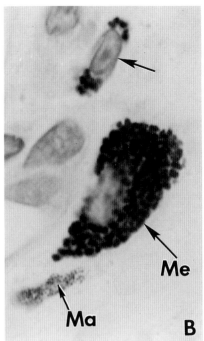
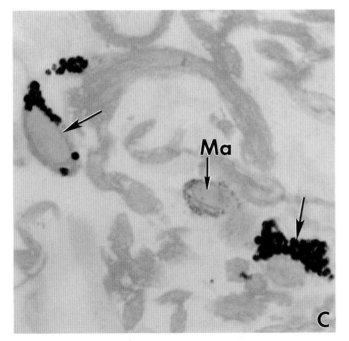
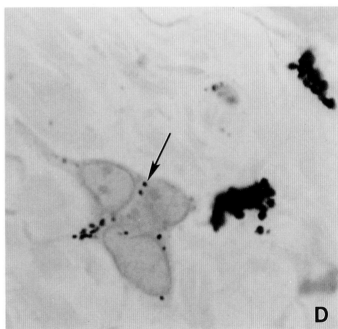

PLATE 52

MULTINUCLEATED GIANT CELLS

Multinucleated giant cells are formed by the fusion of macrophages; their precise function is not known. The presence of multinucleated giant cells is normal in Black skin. They are rare in White skin except in areas that contain hair fragments.

A. Multinucleated giant cells (arrows) in the normal facial skin of a young Black woman. 2-μm plastic section. H and Lee. OM 800x.

B. The cytoplasm of a multinucleated giant cell (arrow) in the face of a middle-aged Black woman has a finely reticulated (foamy) appearance. The small macrophage (M) contains partially degraded melanosomes. 2-μm plastic section. H and Lee. OM 1000x.

C. Cluster of multinucleated giant cells from the normal scalp of a young Black woman. The formation of these cells is associated with the presence of foreign bodies. 2-μm plastic section. H and Lee. OM 1000x.

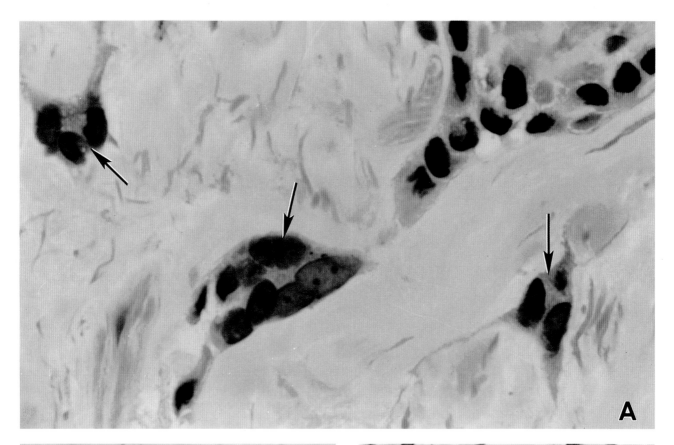

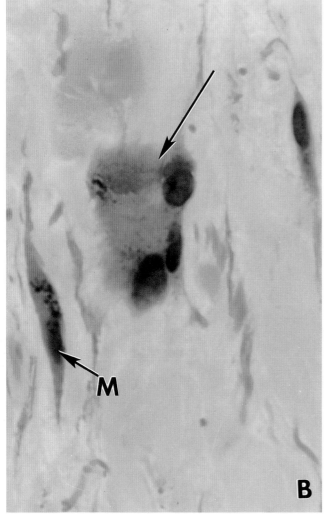

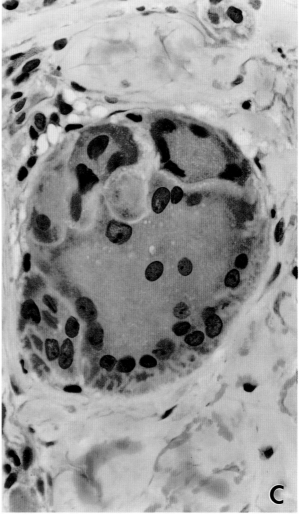

PLATE 53

MACROPHAGES

Macrophages and fibroblasts contain the same metabolic organelles and are similarly located in the dermis; for these reasons, it is sometimes difficult to distinguish a macrophage from a fibroblast. The distinguishing mark of a macrophage is the presence of phagocytic vacuoles. There are different types of macrophages with various structural and functional capabilities.

A. TEM micrograph of a macrophage filled with lysosomes and phagolysosomes (PL) in various stages of development. Membrane-bound vesicles contain hydrolytic enzymes and various other substances synthesized by the macrophages; the contents of the vesicles may be secreted or used in intracellular digestion. Mitochondrion (M). Collagen (C). OM 4500x. Courtesy of Dr. Mary Bell.

B. TEM micrograph of a melanophage, a type of macrophage that degrades melanin. Melanosomes are within phagolysosomes (PL). This macrophage has rough endoplasmic reticulum and Golgi complexes similar to those of fibroblasts, but the phagocytic vacuoles distinguish it from a fibroblast. Mitochondria (M). Collagen (C). OM 5600x.

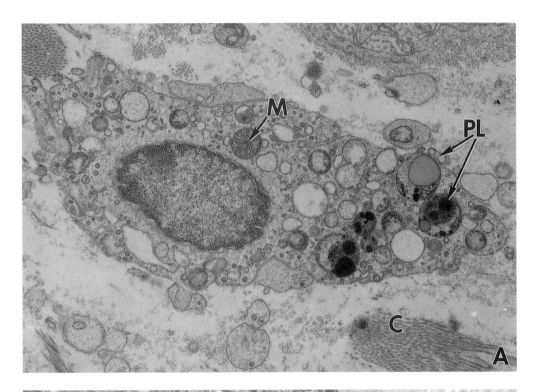

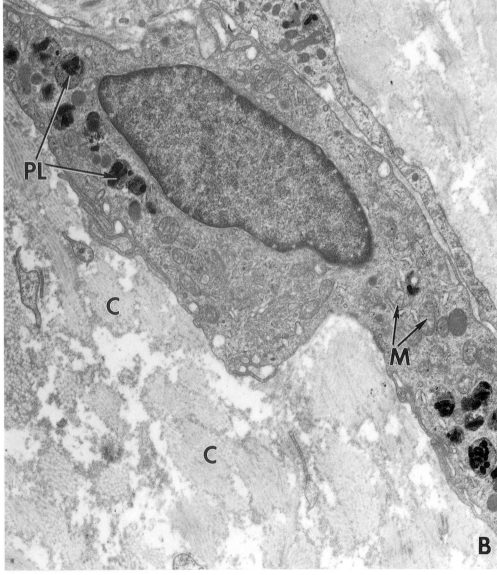

PLATE 54

MAST CELLS

In 1877 a medical student, Paul Ehrlich, discovered granulated dermal cells that stained a metachromatic color with toluidine blue (metachromasia is defined as the staining of a cell or tissue a different color from that of the staining solution). Since he found these cells around blood vessels and assumed that they were feeding, he called them *Mastzellen* (*Mast*, feeding; *Zellen*, cells). We now know that mast cells secrete a variety of substances that influence vascular permeability. Mast cells are numerous in the face, scalp, and external genitalia, tissues that appear to be very active. In contrast, preparations of skin from the trunk, buttock, and extremities, where there appears to be minimal activity, show few mast cells. Various functions have been attributed to mast cells, including vasoactive and smooth muscle-contracting activities, chemotactic factors, proteolysis, and anticoagulation; mast cells participate at each stage of inflammatory reactions whether induced by physical or chemical stimuli. Degranulation of mast cells releases diverse substances that have various functions. Mast cells secrete heparin-like substances, histamine, prostaglandin D_2 (PGD_2), adhesion molecules, leukotrienes, acid hydrolases, and other lytic enzymes.

A. Mast cell granules stain a blue to purplish color in histological sections stained with H and Lee. It is sometimes difficult to identify mast cells without using special stains. 2-μm plastic section. OM 630x.

B. Mast cell granules stain a metachromatic color with toluidine blue. 2-μm plastic section. OM 800x.

C. With the Giemsa stain, mast cell granules are a bright magenta color. 2-μm plastic section. OM 800x.

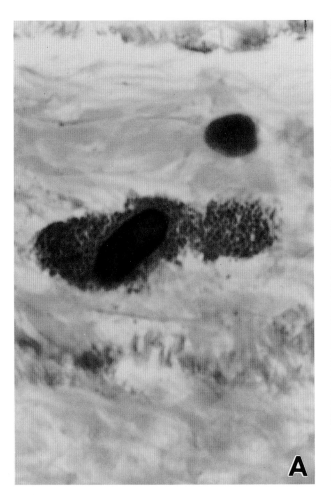

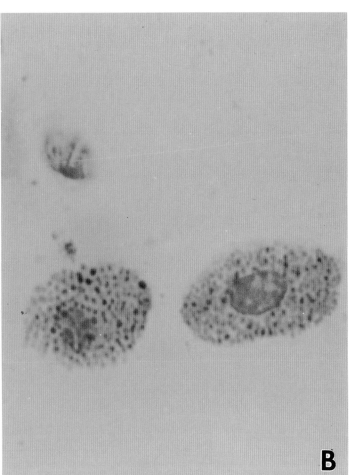

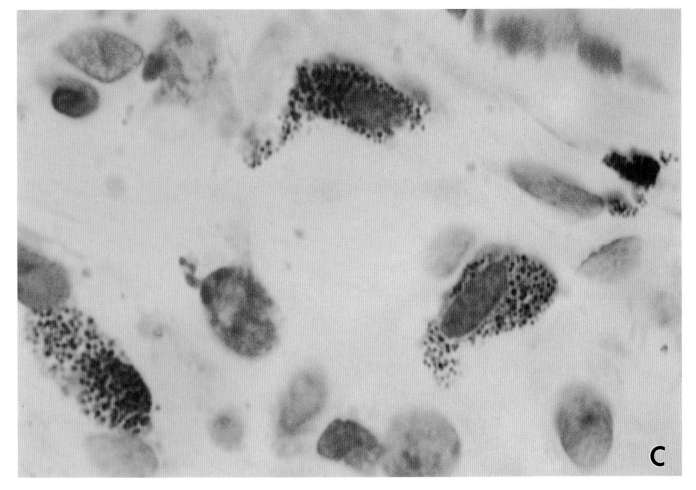

PLATE 55

MAST CELLS

Mast cell granules contain a variety of chemical substances; this may account for the positive reactions with various stains.

A. Mast cell granules stain with Hale's colloidal iron technique for mucopolysaccharides when the staining solution is pH 1.0. From the facial skin of a young woman. 2-μm plastic section. OM 1200x.

B. Mast cell granules from the facial skin of a 4-year-old child stain with Mowry's mucopolysaccharide technique. 2-μm plastic section. OM 1000x.

C. Mast cell granules are Schiff-reactive. 4-μm plastic section. PAS counterstained with hematoxylin. OM 800x.

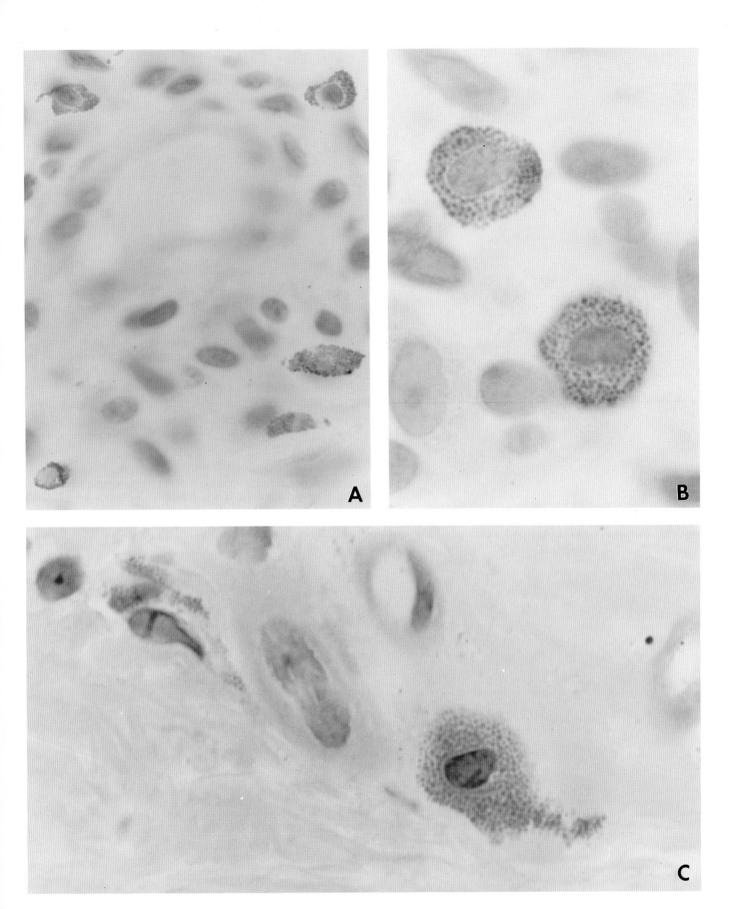

PLATE 56

MAST CELL

TEM micrograph of a dermal mast cell filled with dense granules. Microvilli (M), fine cytoplasmic projections, extend from the cell membrane and increase the surface area of these cells. The plasma membrane of the mast cells can be stimulated by injury, local infection, or immunological reactions. These events trigger the release of the mast cell granules. First the granules fuse, then they attach to the plasma membrane, and finally the contents are extruded into the extracellular space; the response is dependent upon the contents of the granules released. A cytoplasmic portion of another cell (arrow) is in close proximity to the microvilli of the mast cell. Collagen (C). Nucleus (Nu). OM 10,000x.

The inset shows enlarged mast cell granules. The granules have an ordered internal structure with variously arranged lamellae that resemble "scrolls." The granules of mast cells from different body regions have different ultrastructural configurations. OM 52,000x. Courtesy of Dr. Mary Bell.

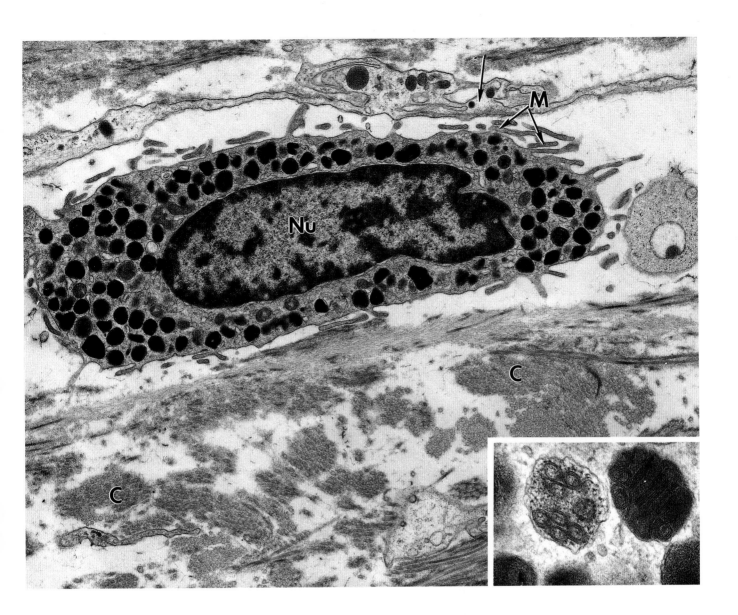

PLATE 57

COLLAGEN and ELASTIC FIBERS

Collagen and elastic fibers are the main types of fibers in the dermis. Collagen makes up 75% of the dry weight of the skin and provides both tensile strength and elasticity. Elastic fibers account for about 4% of the dermal proteins.

Three collagen chains make up a collagen molecule; collagen molecules are crosslinked in the extracellular space into collagen fibrils that can be seen only with an electron microscope. The fibrils collect into small groups or fibers that can be seen with the light microscope. Fibers, in turn, organize into larger fiber bundles. Elastic fibers form a network that borders the collagen bundles.

A. The SEM shows the three-dimensional architecture of the collagen fibers in the dermis. Elastic fibers are intimately intertwined with collagen but cannot be seen in this specimen. Note that the collagen bundles are smaller in the papillary dermis (P) than in the reticular dermis (R), where an elaborate feltwork is formed. OM 160x. Courtesy of Dr. P. Zheng.

B. This SEM micrograph shows the arrangement of elastic tissue in the dermis; the collagen has been removed from the skin by autoclaving. Elastic fibers appear to branch and form a continuous network throughout the dermis. As with collagen, the elastic fibers in the papillary dermis (P) have a smaller diameter than those in the reticular dermis (R). OM 250x. Courtesy of Dr. P. Zheng.

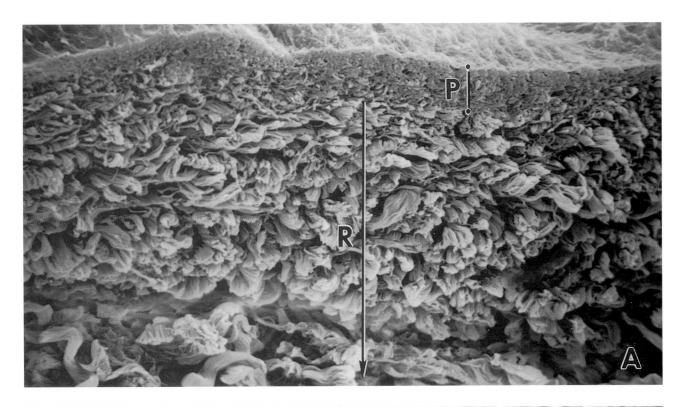

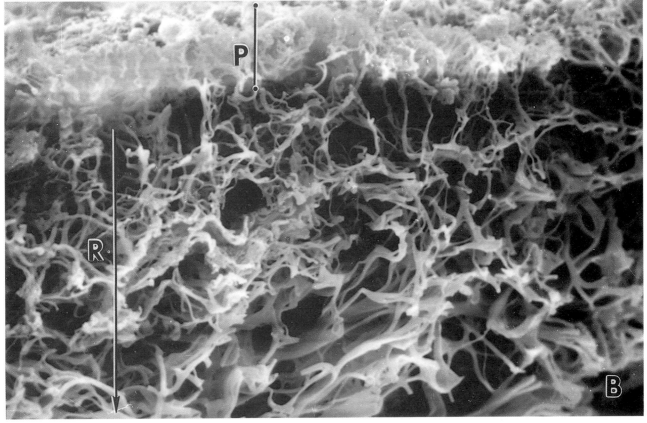

PLATE 58

SURFACE of
PAPILLARY DERMIS

The architecture of the dermal surface after removal of the epidermis from the skin of the chest of a young man. These tufts of papillary dermis consist of small bundles of collagen fibers. The tufts fit inside the "holes" on the underside of the epidermis. These dermal "islands" are distributed around a cone-shaped crater (arrow), which was previously occupied by the acrosyringium of a sweat gland. OM 150x.

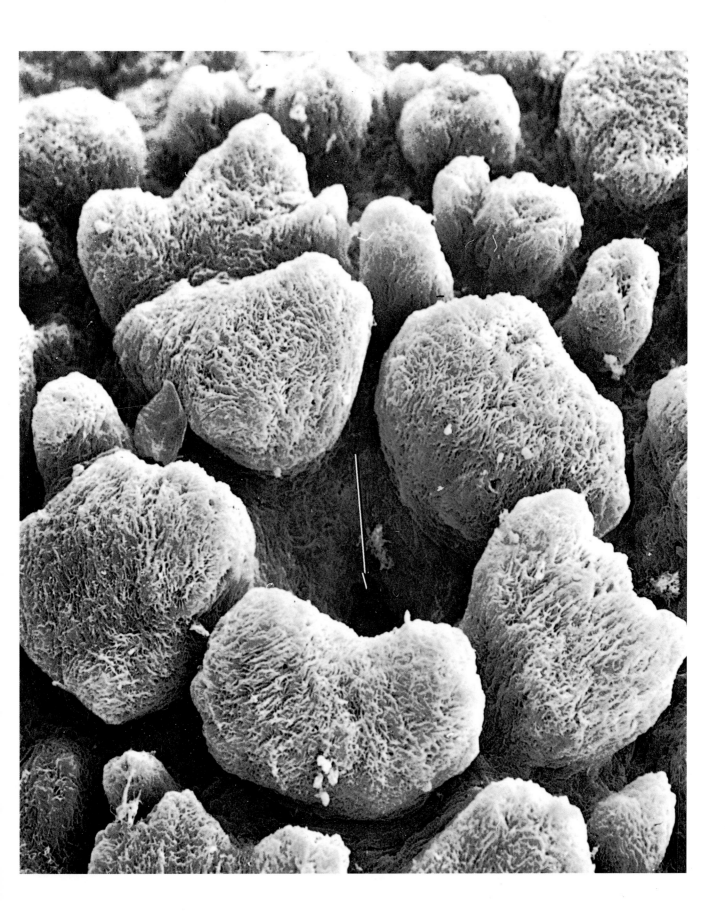

PLATE 59

COLLAGEN FIBERS

The dermis is divided into a papillary layer that follows the contours of the epidermis and a reticular layer that extends from the bottom of the papillary dermis to the hypodermis. The papillary dermis has a high content of type III collagen, which consists of small-diameter fibrils organized into small fiber bundles. Some type I collagen is also present. The reticular dermis is composed primarily of type I collagen, which consists of large-diameter fibrils woven into large fiber bundles. Type I collagen makes up 60 to 80% of the normal adult dermis; about 15 to 20 % is type III collagen. The size of collagenous fibrils and fiber bundles and the ratio of type I to type III collagen in the dermis increase progressively toward the hypodermis.

Under the light microscope, collagen fibers resemble an irregular meshwork. In reality, the fiber bundles are arranged in a somewhat orthogonal pattern; that is, each layer is at right angles to the one above and the one below. These collagen fibers from the facial skin of a young man are stained with a combination of sirius red and sirius blue at pH 1.5. This stain mixture is used because it stains the collagen fibers but not the elastic fibers.

A. Packing of collagenous fiber bundles. The papillary dermis (P) forms a thin band beneath the epidermis (E), and the reticular dermis (R) appears to form a random feltwork. 2-μm plastic section. OM 160x.

Figures B, C, and D are enlargements of regions in Figure A.

B. The papillary dermis (P) in this section is about one-half the thickness of the epidermis (E). Its upper part is composed mostly of very small to small collagenous fiber bundles (1 to 10 μm in width). The fiber bundles tend to be parallel to the surface. These fibers are primarily type III collagen. Note the larger fiber bundles in the upper reticular dermis (R). 2-μm plastic section. OM 630x.

C. The intermediate layer (upper part of the reticular dermis), well defined in the face, consists of small and medium-sized fiber bundles. 2-μm plastic section. OM 630x.

D. In the lower reticular dermis, above the papillae adiposae of the hypodermis, are large collagenous fiber bundles (40+ μm in width) that consist mostly of type I collagen. Smaller collagenous fiber bundles, stained a dark red, are interspersed among the large bundles. 2-μm plastic section. OM 630x.

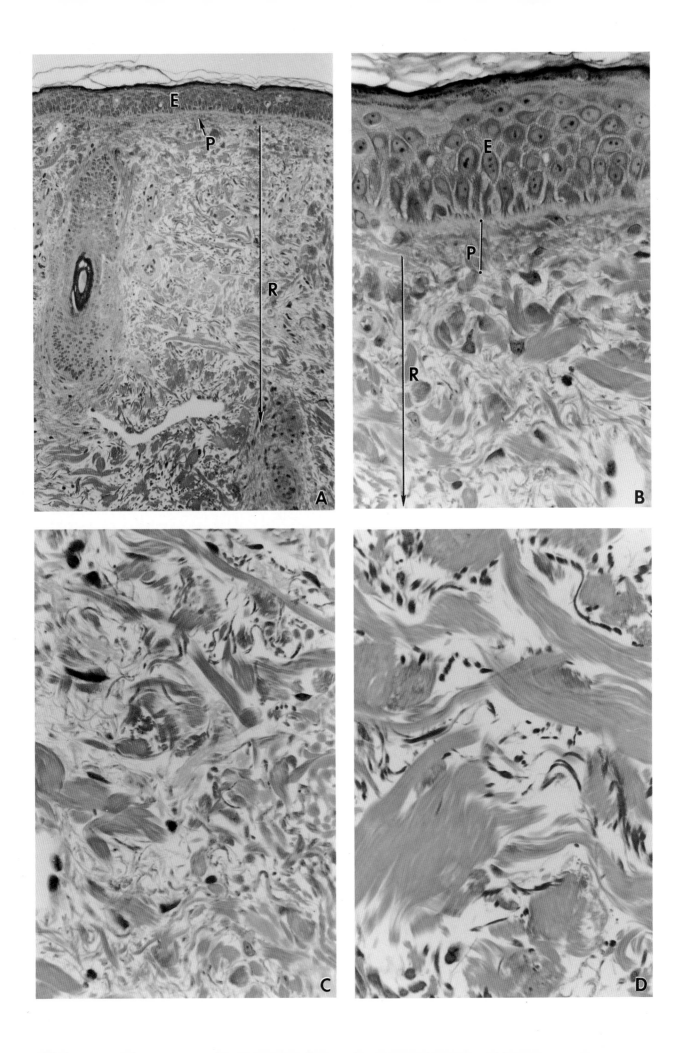

PLATE 60

DERMIS

A. TEM micrograph of the upper reticular dermis. Bundles of collagen fibers (C) are cut in various directions; elastic fibers (E) are scattered among them. The ground substance (GS) of the extracellular matrix, which is known to contain glycosaminoglycans and glycoproteins, appears empty. These molecules interact with the collagen and elastic fibers, and regulate the water-binding capabilities of the dermis. The major glycosaminoglycans in adult skin are hyaluronic acid and dermatin sulfate. Fibronectin, a filamentous glycoprotein in the ground substance, is associated with collagen and elastic fibers and with the basal lamina. Nucleus (N). OM 5000x. Courtesy of Dr. Mary Bell.

B. TEM micrograph of individual collagen fibrils in the dermis of the face of a 20-year-old White woman. An elastic fiber (E) is seen between the longitudinal sections of the banded collagen fibrils (C). The cross sections of collagen fibrils appear as groups of small circles. OM 16,000x. Courtesy of Michael Webb.

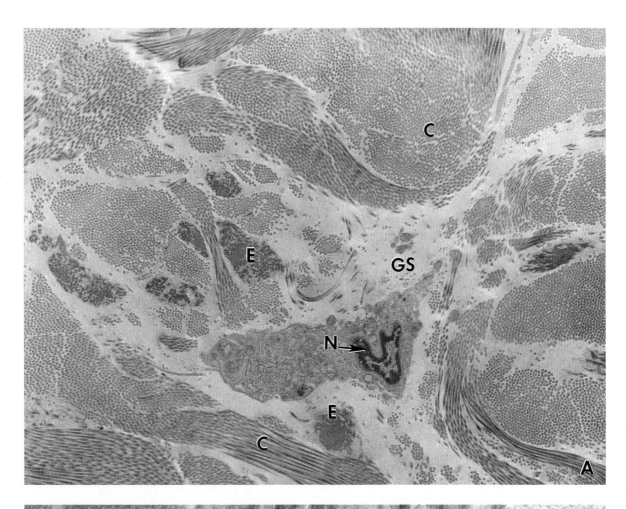

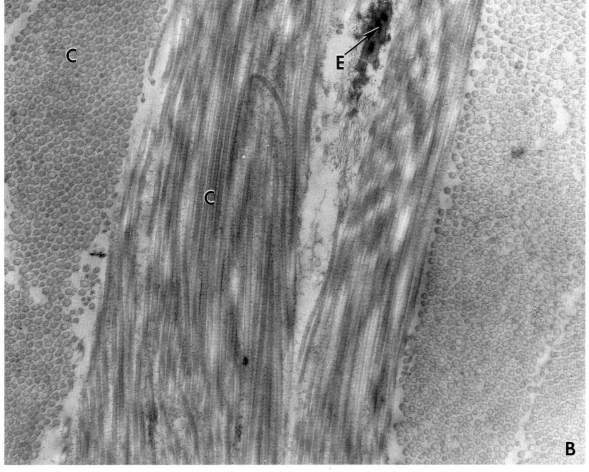

PLATE 61

DERMIS

A. This TEM micrograph from the face of a young Black woman contains cross sections of collagen fibrils (C) and an elastic fiber (E) that consists of an amorphous matrix (A) surrounded by micro-fibrillar material (Mi). The branching, filamentous structures (F) scattered in the extracellular matrix may be glycoprotein molecules. OM 25,000x.

B. Note the dark, dense structures (arrows), which may be cross sections of fine filaments, between the individual collagen fibrils (C) in the face of a Black woman. The identity of these structures is not known; they may be another type of collagen, a glycoprotein, or an elastic component that is intimately associated with the colla-gen fibrils. Fine filamentous structures (F) are numerous in the ma-trix. OM 20,000x.

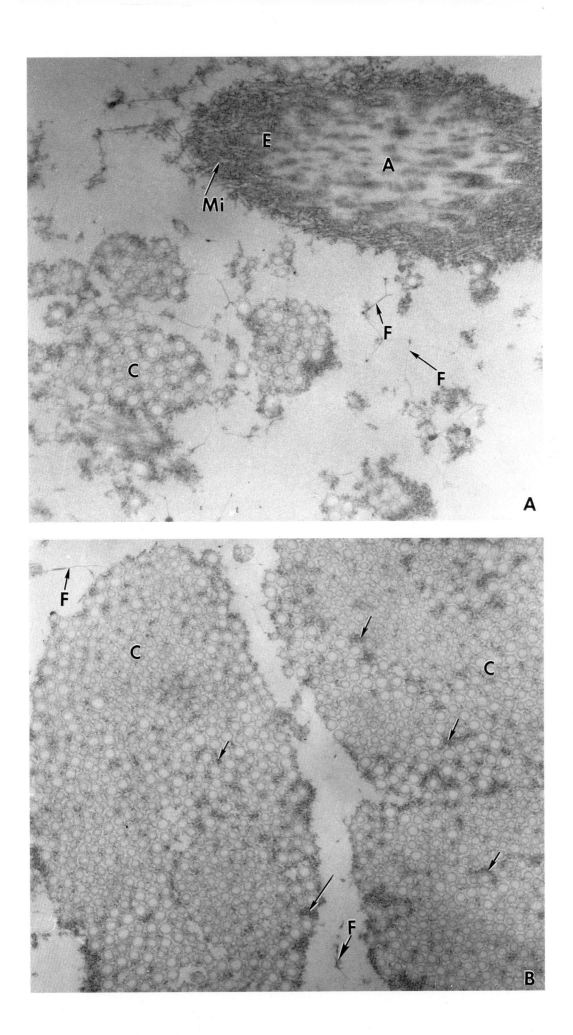

PLATE 62

IMMUNOCYTOCHEMISTRY of COLLAGENS

Immunoelectron microscopic localization of types III and XII collagens associated with the banded collagen fibrils in the dermis.

A. Monoclonal anti-human type III collagen IgM antibody on the surface of collagen fibrils with a periodicity of 67 nm. There is a similar localization on all banded collagen fibrils throughout the dermis. Studies have shown that all banded fibrils in the dermis are composites of type I, type III, and probably also type V collagen. OM 247,000x. Courtesy of Douglas R. Keene and Robert E. Burgeson.

B. Monoclonal anti-human FACIT (Fibril Associated Collagens with Interrupted Triple helices) binds to the surface of the banded collagen fibrils of the dermis. FACIT is believed to include types XII and XIV collagens. This micrograph shows the localization of type XIV collagen on some of the fibrils of a fiber bundle in the papillary dermis from a 20-week fetus. It is thought that the FACIT collagens may be involved in the adhesion of the fibrils. Type XIV collagen appears to be present throughout the reticular dermis, whereas type XII is limited to the papillary dermis. OM 78,000x. Courtesy of Douglas R. Keene and Robert E. Burgeson.

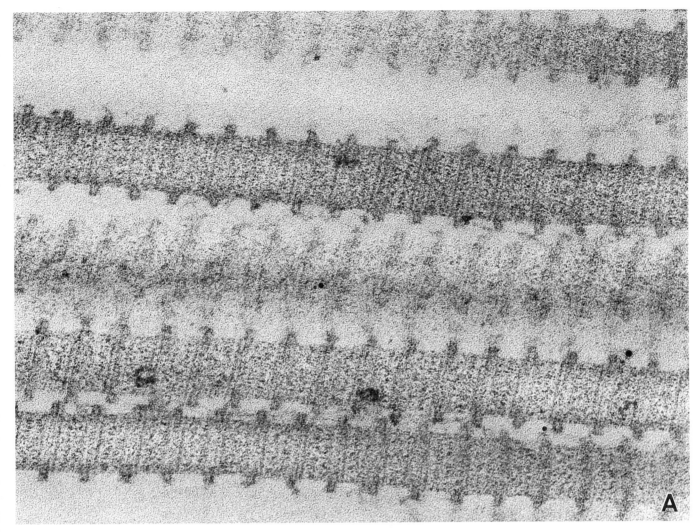

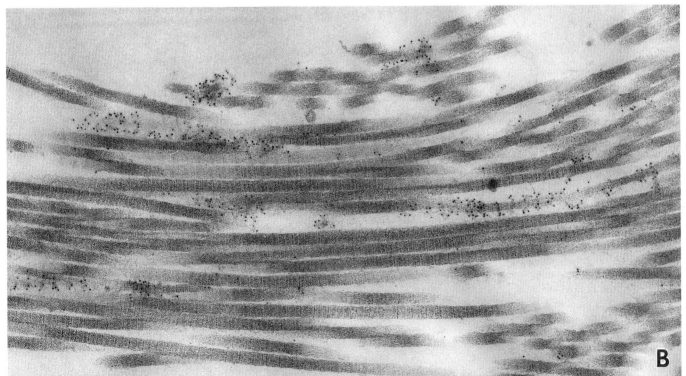

PLATE 63

IMMUNOCYTOCHEMISTRY of COLLAGENS

Immunoelectron microscopic localization of type VI collagen on the beaded filaments surrounding the banded collagen fibrils.

A. SEM micrograph of neonatal foreskin dermis treated with monoclonal anti-human type VI collagen and colloidal gold-conjugated secondary antibody. Type VI collagen forms a fine, independent fiber network that surrounds and binds the fiber bundles. The gnarled appearance of the banded collagenous fibrils is due to the presence of anti-human type III collagen IgM bound on their surfaces. All the fibrils in the field are recognized by the anti-human type III collagen antibody. OM 31,200x. Courtesy of Douglas R. Keene and Robert W. Glanville.

B. TEM micrograph of fibrils in a fiber bundle that was also immunolabeled for type VI collagen. Colloidal gold is deposited on the fine, beaded filaments between the individual fibrils. Beaded filaments in skin are concentrated around blood vessels and nerves. Type VI collagen is believed to form a flexible, web-like network that functions to interrelate the various connective tissue elements while allowing flexibility. From the dermis of a 65-year-old person. OM 101,000x. Courtesy of Douglas R. Keene and Robert W. Glanville. Reproduced from the *Journal of Cell Biology*, 1988, 107: 2001, by copyright permission of the Rockefeller University Press.

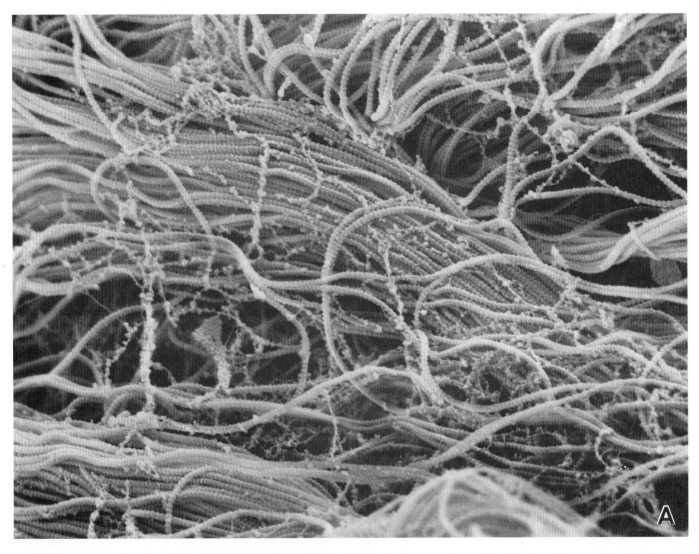

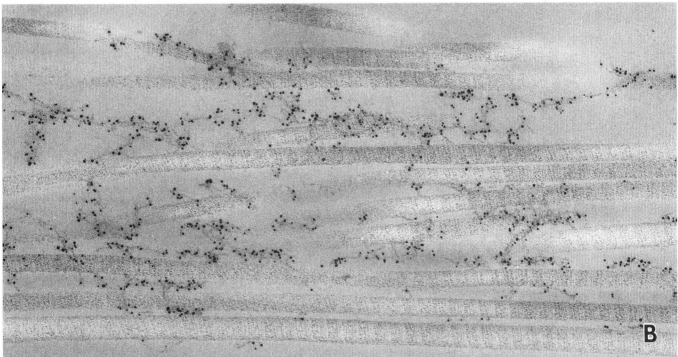

PLATE 64

ELASTIC FIBERS

Elastic fibers make up about 4% of the dry weight of dermal proteins. Some elastic fibers are associated with blood vessels, lymph vessels, hair follicles, eccrine sweat glands, and apocrine glands. They also connect the arrectores pilorum muscles to the bulge region of hair follicles and to their insertion in the papillary dermis.

Mature elastic fibers, elaunin fibers, and oxytalan fibers occur in order of their ascent to the dermal–epidermal junction. Elastic fibers of the skin, like collagenous fibers, become progressively smaller as they ascend toward the epidermis (E). The mature elastic fibers in the lower part of the reticular dermis (R) are thick and stain almost black. Mature elastic fibers consist of microfibrils that are "glued" together with an amorphous elastin matrix. Compare these thick fibers with the thin, terminal elaunin and oxytalan fibers in the papillary dermis (P), which stain a reddish color. The elaunin fibers contain microfibrillar material mixed with a small amount of elastin matrix, and the terminal oxytalan fibers contain only microfibrils. From the axilla of a 55-year-old man. 15-μm frozen section. Roman's AOV elastic fiber technique. OM 120x.

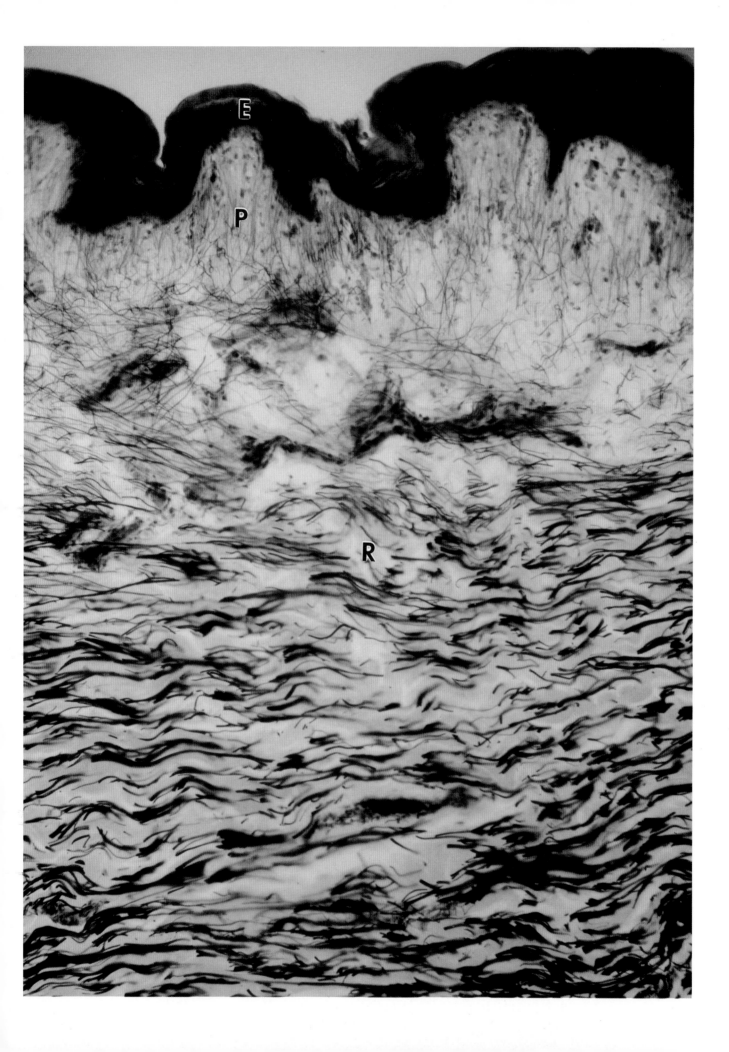

PLATE 65

ELAUNIN and OXYTALAN FIBERS

The architecture of the preterminal and terminal elastic fiber network, also known as elaunin and oxytalan fibers, respectively, is demonstrated in thick (40-μm) frozen sections stained with Roman's AOV elastic fiber technique. There is a similarity in the arrangement of elaunin and oxytalan fibers, regardless of body region.

A. Long elaunin fibers and short, fine oxytalan fibers in the nipple of the well-developed breast of a 14-year-old girl. OM 375x.

B. Moderately long oxytalan fibers from the chest of a 25-year-old man. OM 400x.

C. The elaunin fibers in the finger of a 57-year-old man form a matted layer from which short oxytalan fibers rise to the epidermis. OM 375x.

D. Subepidermal elastic fibers in the glabella of a 55-year-old man. The elastic network is very dense and matted, probably reflecting photodamage in this exposed region. The skin of the face normally contains large amounts of elastic tissue. OM 400x.

E. Long oxytalan fibers are characteristic of axillary skin. From the axilla of a 53-year-old man. OM 400x.

F. Well-developed subepidermal elastic fibers from the axilla of a 6-month-old boy resemble those in Figure E. OM 400x.

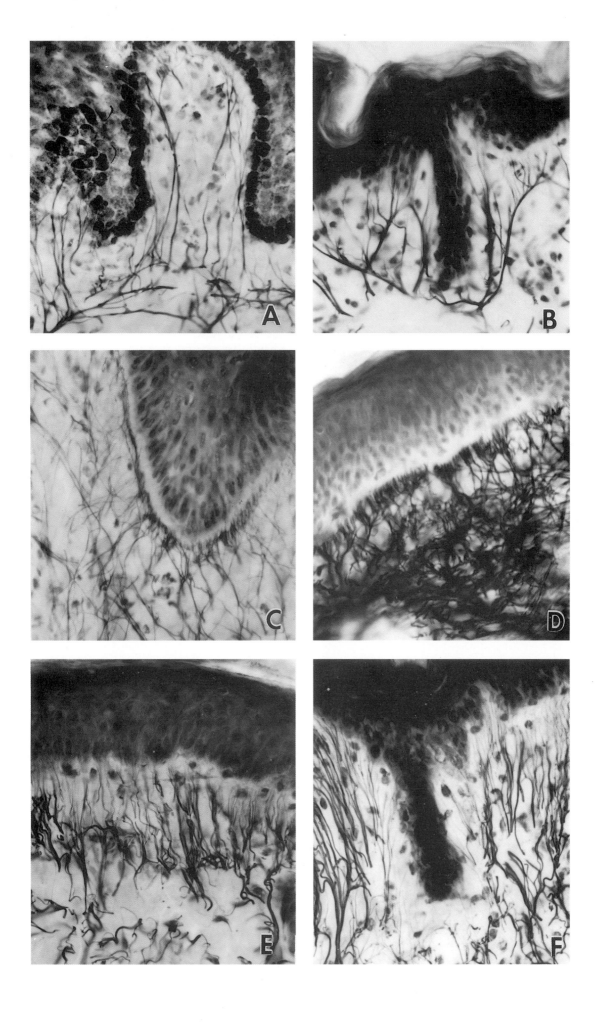

PLATE 66

ELASTIC FIBERS

A. Elaunin (En) and oxytalan (O) fibers in the papillary body of the chest. Mature elastic fibers (Ea) run parallel to the skin surface. The elaunin fibers terminate in two distinct patterns. On the left and right of the blood vessel (BV), the fibers come together and form a coarse brush-like matting (arrows), while the elaunin fibers in the center send long branches upward. Fine, delicate oxytalan fibers branch from the elaunin fibers and travel directly toward the base of the epidermis; they lose their stainability before reaching the basement membrane. Mixed patterns of elastic fiber termination are common in human skin. The function of these fibers is to anchor the epidermis to the dermis. 40-μm frozen section. Roman's AOV elastic fiber technique. OM 250x.

B. Section through the reticular dermis of the scalp. The different-sized elastic fibers resemble branching ribbons (arrow). The thickest elastic fibers measure about 5 μm in width. 30-μm frozen section. Roman's AOV elastic fiber technique. OM 250x.

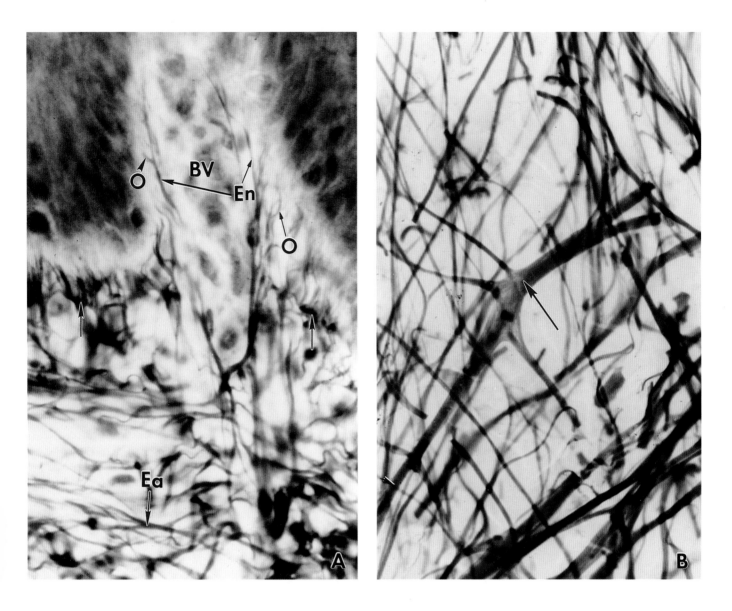

PLATE 67

ELASTIC FIBERS

The architecture of the elastic fiber network differs in Black and White skin.

A. The skin of the face of a young White man with a modest amount of elastosis; note the photodamaged, vacuolated epidermis. The elastic fibers in the upper reticular dermis (RD) are thick, curled, and branched. The exposed skin of White persons shows abnormal elastic fibers (elastosis) in their teens. Papillary dermis (PD). 2-μm plastic section. Weigert's elastic fiber technique. OM 250x.

B. Very fine elastic fibers (arrows) throughout the dermis in the facial skin of a 45-year-old Black woman. There appears to be no elastosis; melanin and other components in Black skin protect the elastic fibers from photodamage. Papillary dermis (PD). Reticular dermis (RD). 4-μm plastic section. Weigert's elastic fiber technique. OM 250x.

C. The elaunin (E) and oxytalan (O) fibers, from the face of a 20-year-old White woman, which make up the terminal portion of the elastic network in the papillary dermis, resemble inverted candelabra. The elastic fibers directly below the terminal fibers are thickened and branched. 2-μm plastic section. Weigert's elastic fiber technique. OM 630x.

D. Long, thin oxytalan fibers (O) rise up from short elaunin fibers (E) in Black facial skin; this distribution of elastic fibers is characteristic of Black facial skin. Compare the pattern of terminal fibers in the Black skin with that of the White skin in Figure C. 2-μm plastic section. Weigert's elastic fiber technique. OM 630x.

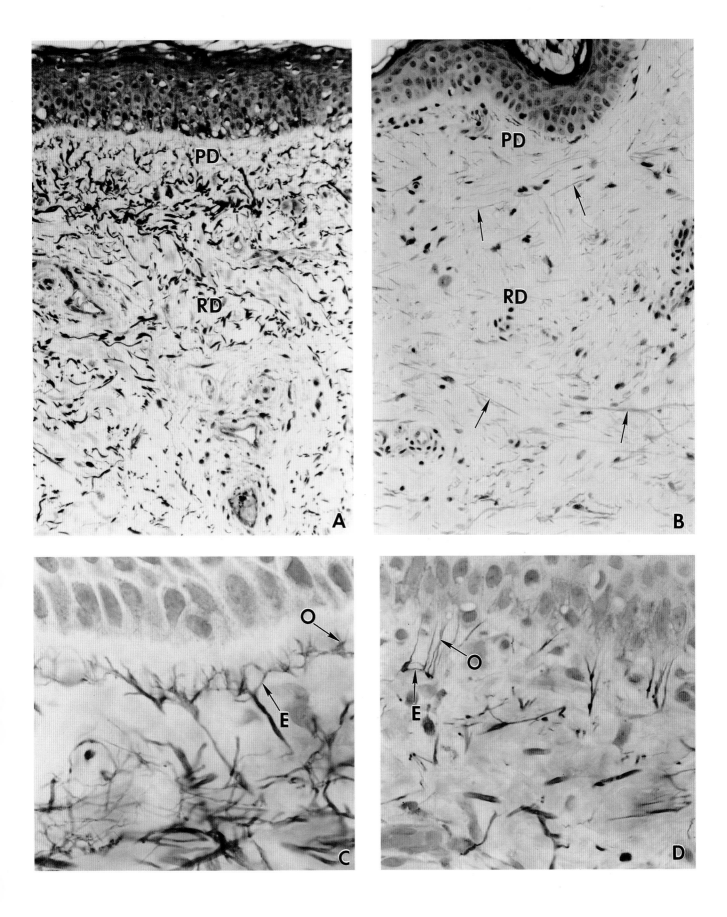

PLATE 68

ELASTIC FIBERS
Aging

A. SEM micrograph of the elastic fiber network of the photo-damaged dorsal forearm. In photoaged skin, the elastic fibers are thick, highly curled, and branched even in the papillary dermis (P). The collagen fibers have been removed by autoclaving. Reticular dermis (R). OM 250x. Courtesy of Dr. P. Zheng.

B. SEM micrograph of the elastic fiber feltwork in the papillary dermis of the skin of the abdomen of a young adult person. The fibers are thin in the papillary body (P), and both thick and thin in the reticular dermis (R). Autoclave technique. OM 320x. Courtesy of Dr. P. Zheng.

C. Elastic fiber network in the skin of the abdomen of an elderly person shows an increased quantity of curled elastic fibers, an age-dependent phenomenon, even in protected skin. Papillary dermis (P). Reticular dermis (R). Autoclave technique. OM 320x. Courtesy of Dr. P. Zheng.

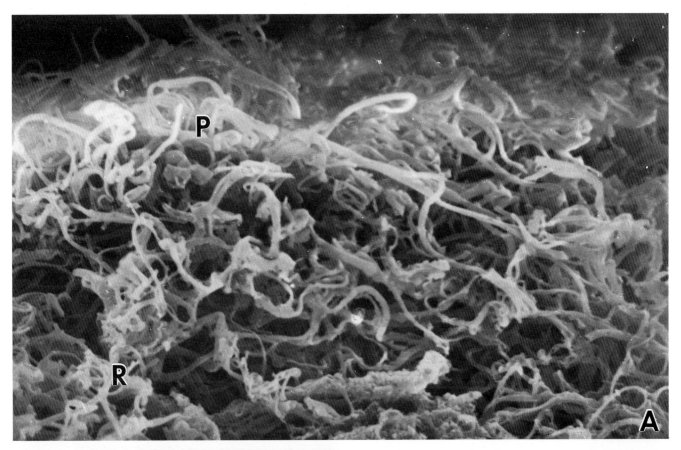

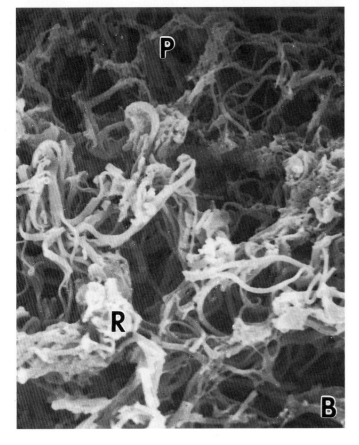

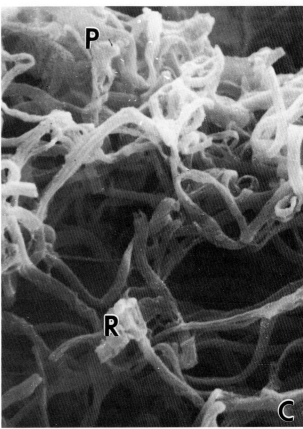

PLATE 69

ELASTIC FIBERS

A. SEM micrograph of an elastic fiber (E) consisting of an amorphous elastin core surrounded by a sheath of microfibrils (Mi) that give the fiber shape and direction. Both components are synthesized by fibroblasts, as are the neighboring collagenous fiber bundles (C). Courtesy of Lynn Y. Sakai and Douglas R. Keene.

B. TEM micrograph of an elastic fiber. The dense particles (arrows) on the periphery of the amorphous elastin core (A) indicate the presence of a monoclonal antibody specific for "fibrillin," a major component of microfibrils. Courtesy of Lynn Y. Sakai and Douglas R. Keene.

C. Elastic fibers are connected to the dermal–epidermal junction by bundles of microfibrils (arrows) known as oxytalan fibers. The microfibrils encircle the amorphous core of the mature elastic fiber in the reticular dermis, travel through the papillary dermis, and eventually intersect the lamina densa of the basal lamina (BL). Courtesy of Lynn Y. Sakai and Douglas R. Keene.

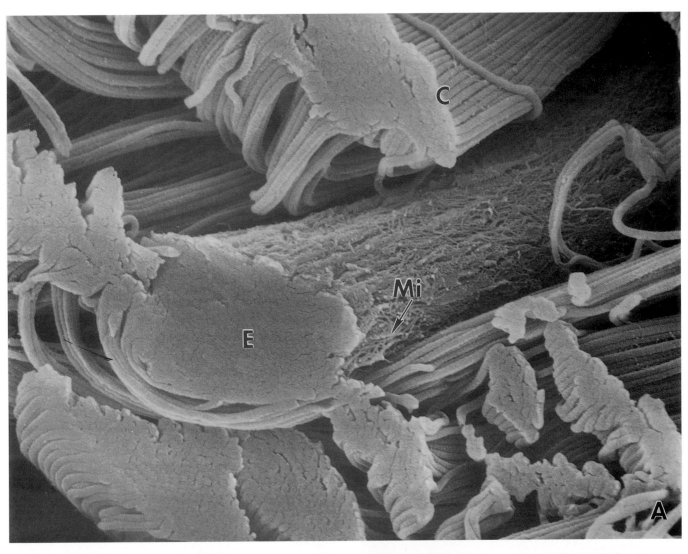

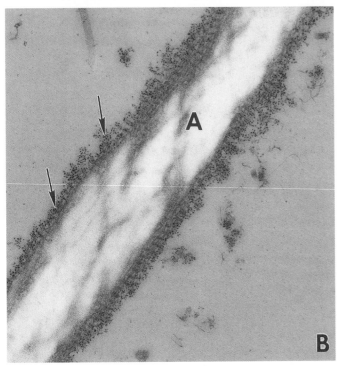

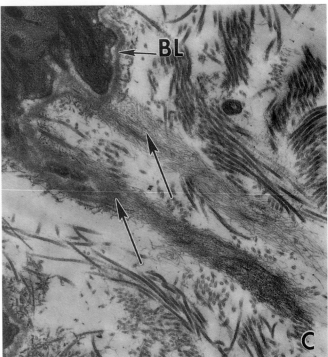

PLATE 70

DERMIS

Minimal Photodamage

These three sections of facial skin from a 35-year-old White man are treated with different stains to show cellular detail, collagen fibers, and elastic fibers. This man used sunscreen daily for many years; there is minimal photodamage. Compare these photographs with those on the next plate, which show severely photodamaged skin.

A. Both the epidermis (Ep) and the dermis (D) are in good condition. Large fibroblasts are scattered among the pale-pink-stained collagenous fibers and red-stained elastic fibers (El) in the dermis. Blood vessels and lymph vessels appear to be normal. 2-μm plastic section. H and Lee. OM 160x.

B. This section shows that collagen fiber bundles (stained pinkish-red) are well packed and distributed throughout the dermis. The fibers become progressively larger as they descend from the papillary dermis (P) through the reticular dermis (R). Note that the epidermal granular layer and the compact stratum lucidum also stain red. Epidermis (Ep). 2-μm plastic section. Sirius red. OM 160x.

C. This section was stained for elastic fibers. The oxytalan and elaunin fibers under the epidermis (Ep) are very fine and well delineated. The elastic fibers of the reticular dermis tend to run parallel to the epidermis; there is minimal elastosis. 4-μm plastic section. Weigert's elastic fiber technique. OM 160x.

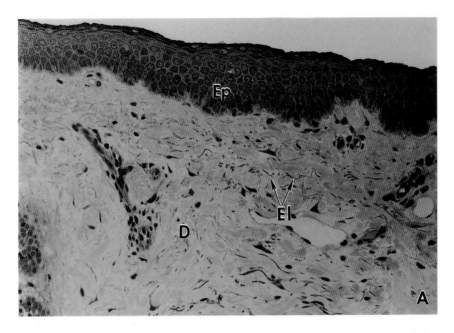

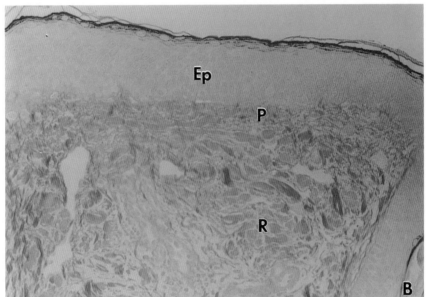

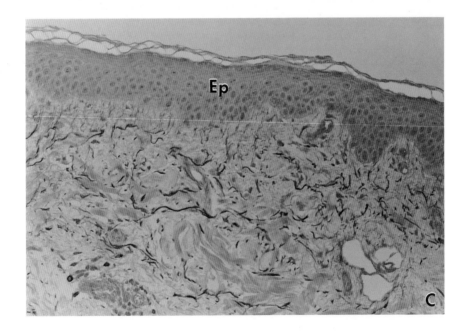

PLATE 71

DERMIS
Photodamage

Excessive exposure of skin to sunlight results in photodamage. All exposed White skin, as early as adolescence, shows some photodamage. After decades of exposure to sun and other environmental hazards, gross damage persists, especially in the dermis where the resorption of damaged fibers may require long periods of time.

These serial sections of facial skin from a 70-year-old sun lover are treated with three different stains that show the combined effects of photoaging and chronological aging on cells, collagen fibers, and elastic fibers. Reproduced with permission of Richardson-Vicks, a Procter and Gamble Company, from: Montagna, Carlisle and Kirchner, *Epidermal and Dermal Histological Markers of Photodamaged Human Facial Skin.* 1989.

A. Both the epidermis (Ep) and the dermis are severely damaged. The epidermal cells are vacuolated and show a great amount of atypia. The stratum lucidum (L) is swollen. The dermis is elastotic and contains round, amorphous masses (A) and twisted, abnormal, pink-staining elastic fiber fragments. There is a very thin Grenz zone (G) just under the epidermis. The rectangular empty space is a telangiectatic vessel (V). 2-μm plastic section. H and Lee. OM 160x.

B. The absence of staining in the mid-dermis shows that the bundles of collagen (C) have largely disappeared. Only a few reddish-pink-stained collagenous fibers remain in the upper dermis near the Grenz zone (G). The thickened stratum lucidum (L) of the epidermis (Ep) indicates severe photodamage. Vessel (V). 2-μm plastic section. Sirius red. OM 160x.

C. Most of the dermis in this section consists of vastly increased, disorganized elastotic material due to severe photodamage. Only a few large, pale-stained collagenous fibers (arrows) can be seen scattered in the mass of elastotic material. Epidermis (Ep). 4-μm plastic section. Weigert's elastic fiber technique. OM 160x.

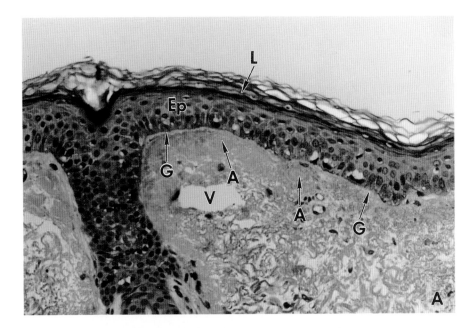

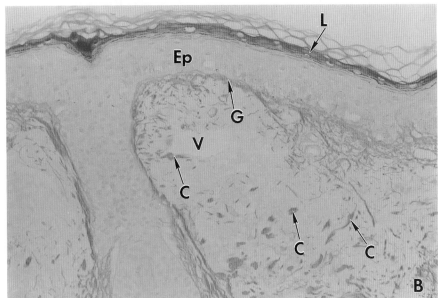

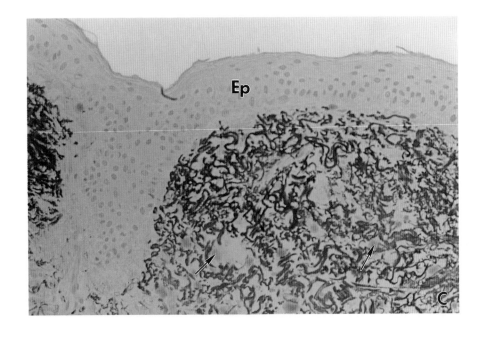

PLATE 72

ELASTIC FIBERS
Photodamage

A. In normal skin, all elastic fibers (E) in the papillary, intermediate, and reticular dermis stain a pink color with H and Lee. The collagenous fibers (C) stain a very pale mauve color. From the face of a young woman. 2-μm plastic section. H and Lee. OM 400x.

B. After chronic exposure to sunlight, the pink elastic fibers (E) in the upper reticular dermis become lysed, fragmented, and show blue-staining longitudinal striations when stained with H and Lee. The nature of the blue-staining striations and fragments is not known. The collagenous fibers (C) are pale-colored. 2-μm plastic section. H and Lee. OM 400x.

C. The bluish-purple-staining elastic fibers (E) in the intermediate layer of the reticular dermis of the facial skin of a young White woman are the first indices of photodamage. (In the skin of Black persons, these ribbon-like fibers continue to stain dark pink, even after long exposure to sunlight.) Note the contrast in staining quality between the elastic fibers and the collagenous fibers (C). 2-μm plastic section. H and Lee. OM 400x.

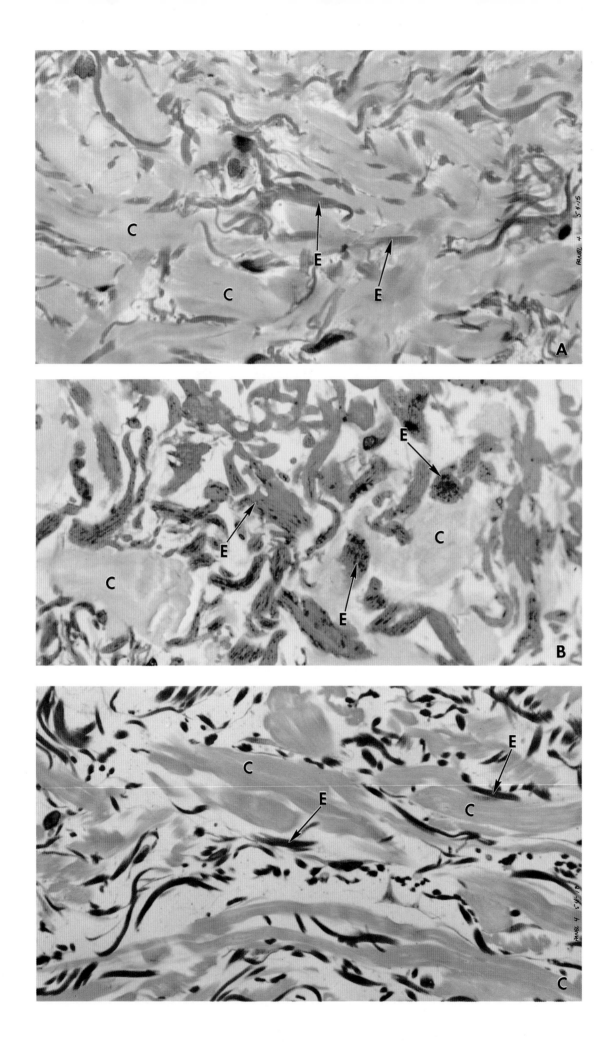

PLATE 73

DERMAL FIBROLYSIS

A. Fibrolysis and fibrorhexis are present in the papillary dermis of this severely photodamaged facial skin of a young White woman The pink-staining, thickened, and twisted elastotic fibers are indicators of photodamage. Rounded, amorphous masses (A), also called elastin globes of Pinkus, are end stages of elastolysis. 2-μm plastic section. H and Lee. OM 400x.

B. In this severely photodamaged face of a young White woman, there is massive destruction of collagen and elastin. There are small, lilac-colored, amorphous masses (A) and a larger mass (LA) stained pink that represent areas in which the elastic fibrous components of the dermis are undergoing lysis. The cells (arrow) attached to this large, amorphous elastotic mass are probably macrophages. 2-μm plastic section. H and Lee. OM 400x.

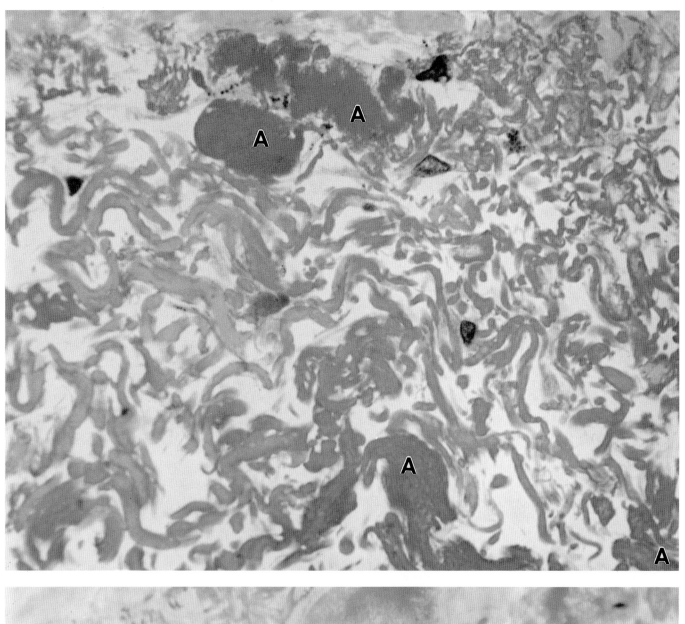

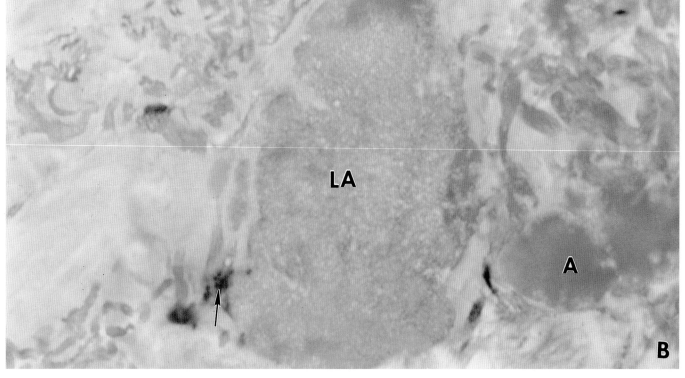

Blood Vessels

The skin has a rich supply of blood and lymph vessels that are nutritive as well as important in the regulation of temperature and blood pressure. The kinds of cutaneous vascular beds present are determined by the kinds of skin they perfuse, the types and numbers of appendages present, and the thickness of the dermal and hypodermal layers. Everywhere on the human body skin is vascularized by vessels that greatly exceed the need for nutrition.

PLATE 74

MICROVASCULATURE

Diagram and Reconstruction

A. Human skin has a blood supply that is greatly in excess of its nutritive needs. This schematic drawing of the cutaneous microcirculation shows ascending arterioles entering the subcutaneous fat. They rise up to the dermis, branch off horizontally, and form a plexus, as well as sending branches to hair follicles and sweat glands. In the papillary dermis, ascending arterioles divide into smaller arterioles that form a superficial vascular plexus oriented parallel to the surface of the skin. Vessels from this plexus divide into smaller terminal arterioles, the ascending or afferent limb of the capillary loops. Postcapillary venules, the descending or efferent limbs of the capillary loops, are the collecting system of the capillaries that empty into the venules of the superficial venular plexus. The venous blood from the superficial venular plexus then empties into descending collecting venules that return the blood to the systemic circulation. From O. T. Tan and T. J. Stafford. In Fitzpatrick, Eisen, Wolff, Freedberg, and Austen *Dermatology in General Medicine (3rd Ed.)*. page 358. Reproduced with permission of McGraw-Hill, Inc.

B. Computer reconstruction of the vessels in 2-mm-wide and 0.67-mm-thick normal human thoracic skin. Zones 1 and 2 contain the dermal capillary loops, and zones 2 and 3 contain vessels of the horizontal plexus. Ascending arteriole (A) with five branches. The accompanying descending venule (V) is formed by converging postcapillary venules. The arrows indicate the capillary loops in the dermal papillae. Epidermis (E). Reprinted by permission of Elsevier Science Publishing Co., Inc. from Correlation of Laser Doppler Wave Patterns, by I. M. Braverman, A. Keh, and D. Golminz in *Journal of Investigative Dermatology* 95:285. Copyright 1990 by the Society for Investigative Dermatology, Inc.

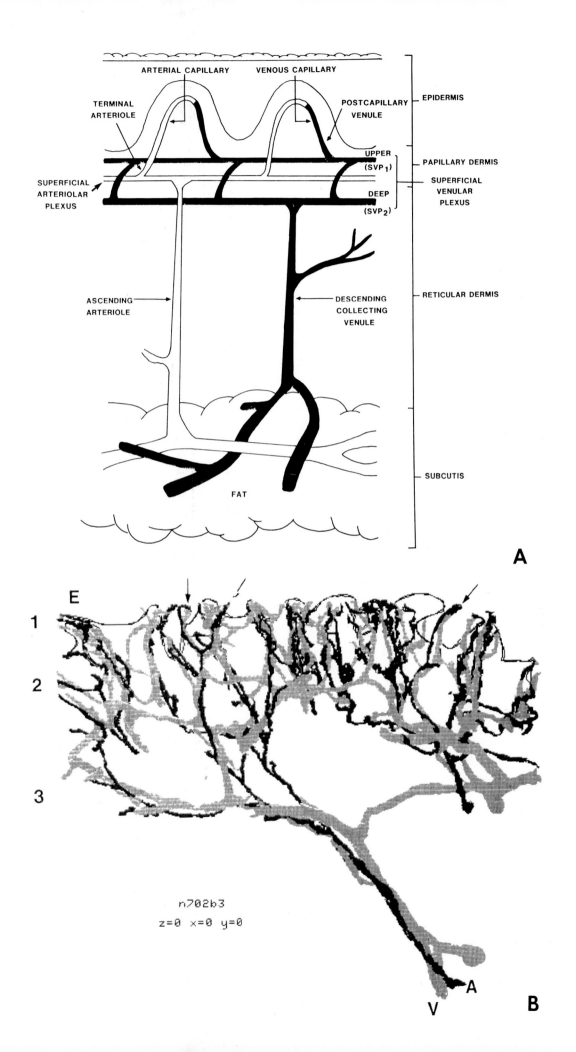

ARTERIAL CAPILLARY   VENOUS CAPILLARY

TERMINAL
ARTERIOLE

POSTCAPILLARY
VENULE

EPIDERMIS

UPPER
(SVP₁)

PAPILLARY DERMIS

SUPERFICIAL
ARTERIOLAR
PLEXUS

SUPERFICIAL
VENULAR
PLEXUS

DEEP
(SVP₂)

ASCENDING
ARTERIOLE

DESCENDING
COLLECTING
VENULE

RETICULAR DERMIS

SUBCUTIS

FAT

A

E

1

2

3

n702b3

z=0 x=0 y=0

A

V

B

PLATE 75

VASCULARITY
Face

The histology of the skin's vascular system reflects its nutritive and thermal functions. There are a number of blood vessels in this facial skin of a 65-year-old Black woman. Note the distribution of the blood and lymph vessels of the subpapillary plexus (P). Lymph vessels (L) with valves are present in both mid- and lower reticular dermis. Ascending arterioles and descending venules are located in the reticular dermis. There is a sebaceous gland acinus (S) surrounded by small vessels at the bottom, near the papillae adiposae of the hypodermis (H). Observe further that this skin specimen, from the facial skin of an older Black woman, has minimal photodamage. 4-μm plastic section. Verhoff's elastic fiber technique. OM 160x.

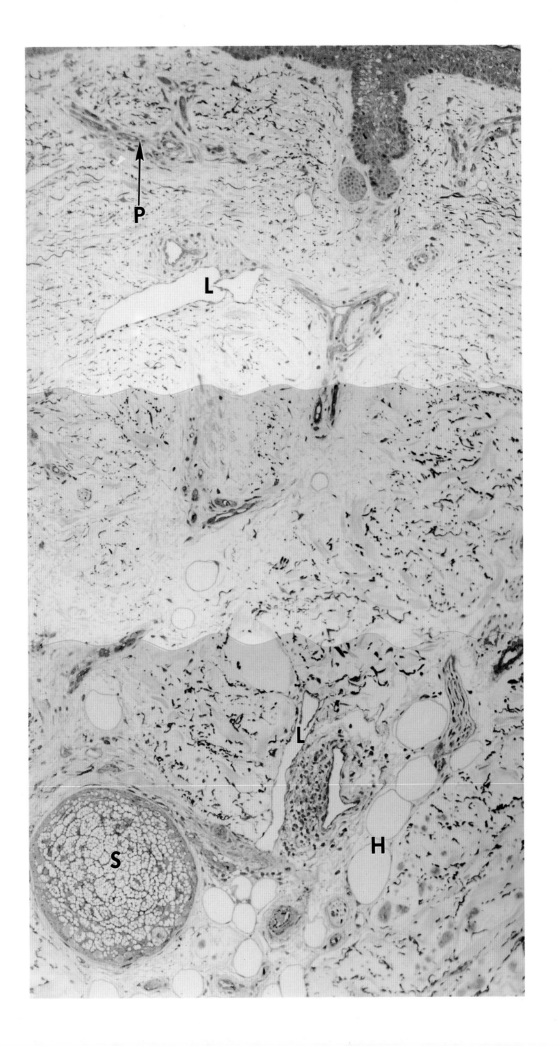

PLATE 76

VASCULARITY

Axilla and Lip

A. Cutaneous vascular elements vary with the kind of skin they perfuse and the types and numbers of skin appendages present. This axillary skin of a 21-year-old man contains many capillary loops and vessels deeper in the dermis. 20-μm frozen section. Gomori's alkaline phosphatase technique. OM 70x.

B. The microvasculature of the lip of an 8-month fetus shows the transition (arrow) from the vermilion border on the right to the mucous portion on the left. Thick epidermis is always supplied by taller and more complex superficial capillary loops than thinner epidermis. 30-μm frozen section. Gomori's alkaline phosphatase technique. OM 100x.

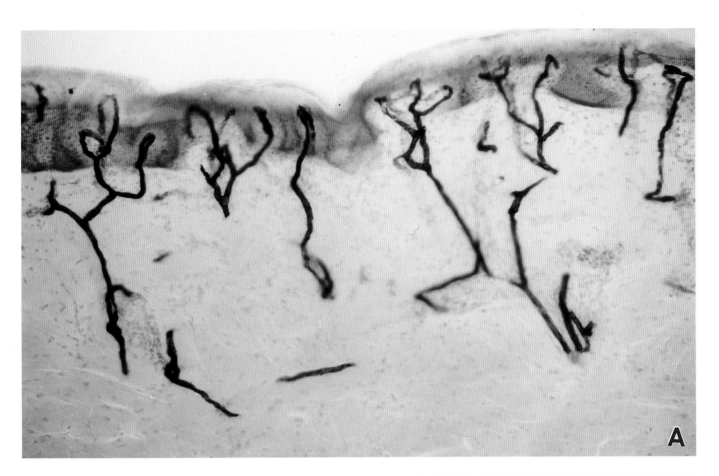

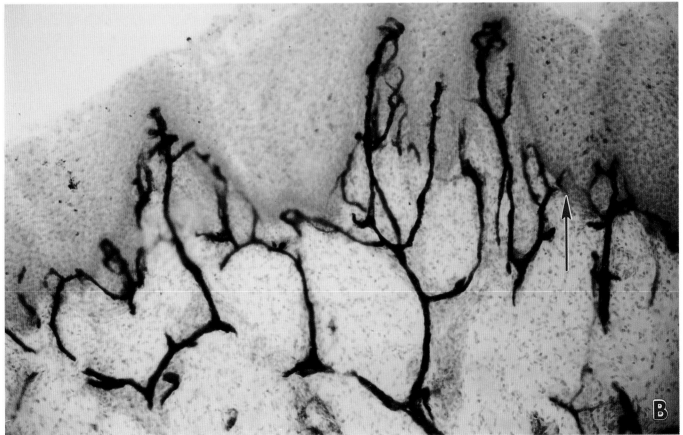

PLATE 77

VASCULARITY

Ears

A. The rich microvasculature of the external ears is primarily a means of thermoregulation. This section from the helix of the ear of a 28-year-old man shows that the arterioles (A) have a stronger reaction for alkaline phosphatase than the venules (V). 30-μm frozen section. Gomori's alkaline phosphatase technique. OM 125x.

B and C. Intricate capillary loops in the earlobe of a 20-year-old man. There are many shunts (S) between the ascending arterioles (A) and the descending venules (V). The ascending arterioles are thinner and stain more intensely than the descending venules. 20-μm frozen section. Gomori's alkaline phosphatase technique. OM 250x.

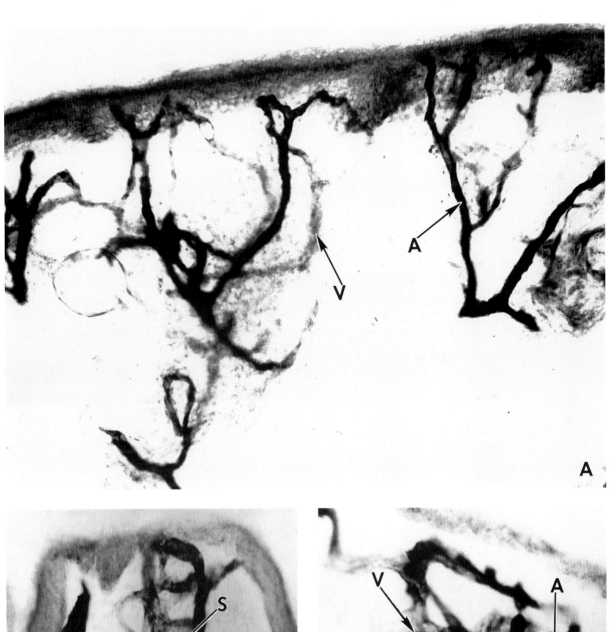

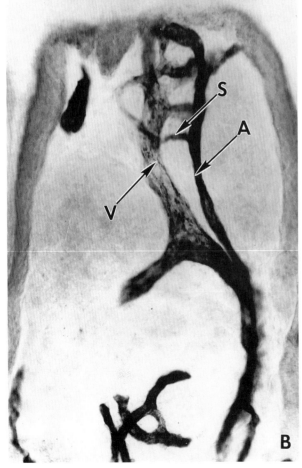

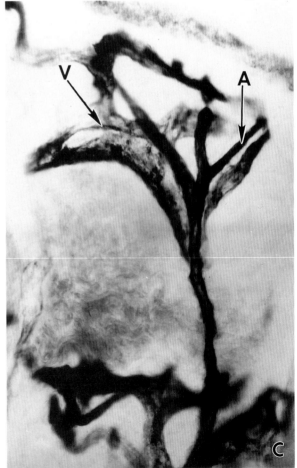

PLATE 78

VASCULARITY
Eyelid

A. The blood vessels in the inner surface of the eyelids form a rich capillary meshwork inside the conjunctiva; thick sections (30 μm) are necessary to appreciate the architecture of the microvasculature. These numerous vessels reflect the high metabolic activity of the conjunctiva. 30-μm frozen section. Gomori's alkaline phosphatase technique. OM 50x.

B. Enlarged detail of the elaborate superficial vascular plexus in the conjunctival blood vessels from Figure A. 30-μm frozen section. Gomori's alkaline phosphatase technique. OM 250x.

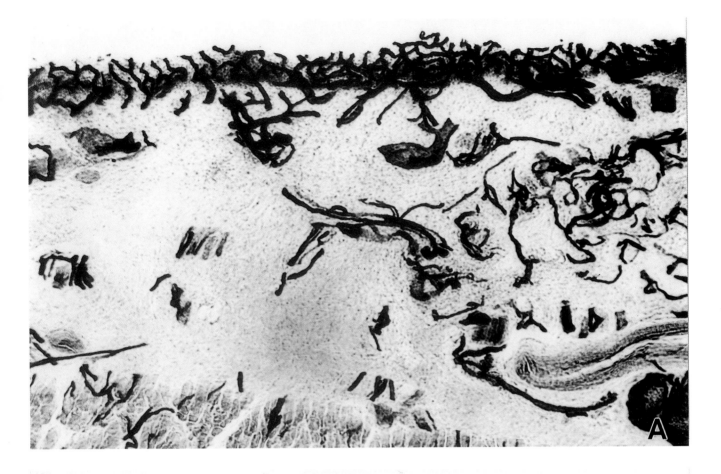

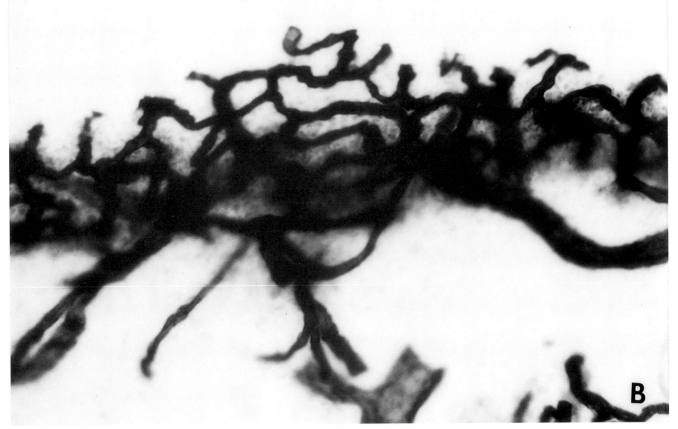

PLATE 79

VASCULARITY
Aging Changes

Cervix

A. Capillary loops are elaborate under the thick epidermis of the cervix of a 20-year-old woman; note the cross shunts at the tips, which enable greater blood flow. The loops empty into venules. 20-μm frozen section. Gomori's alkaline phosphatase technique. OM 50x.

B. With advancing age, the microvasculature of the cervix undergoes degenerative changes that impair function. These capillary loops in the cervix of a 72-year-old woman are shortened, swollen, and distorted. 20-μm frozen section. Gomori's alkaline phosphatase technique. OM 50x.

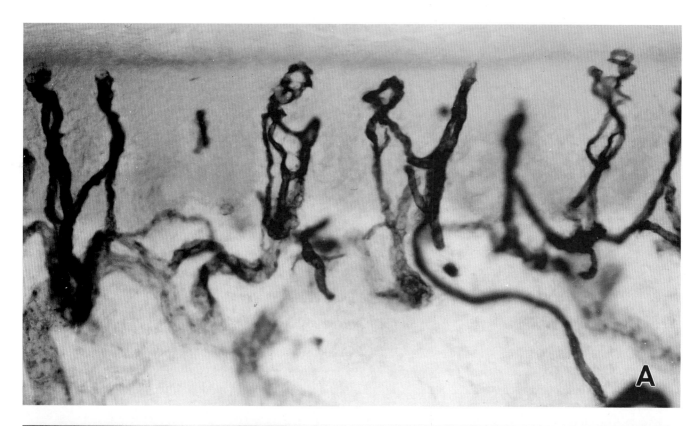

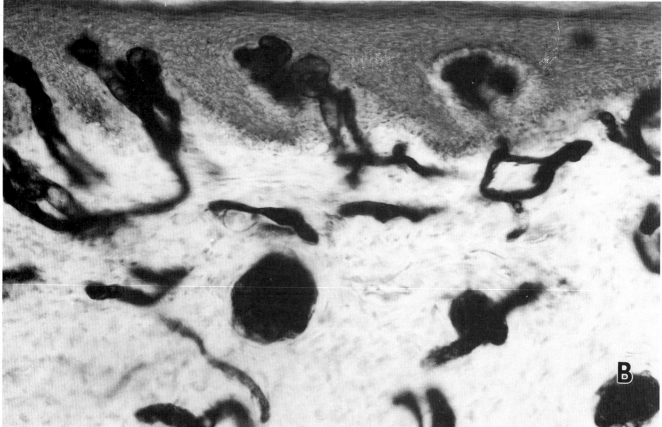

PLATE 80

VASCULARITY
Finger

A. Finger skin with many vessels, from a young man. In areas where the rete ridges are well developed, vascular loops are numerous, elaborate, and so near the epidermis that their individual basement membranes appear to fuse (arrowheads). This arrangement facilitates diffusion of nutrients to the epidermis. The precapillary arterioles (A) are prominent. 4-μm plastic section. PAS lightly counterstained with hematoxylin. OM 250x.

B. Capillary loops in the papillary dermis in the finger skin of a young man. 30-μm frozen section. Gomori's alkaline phosphatase technique. OM 100x.

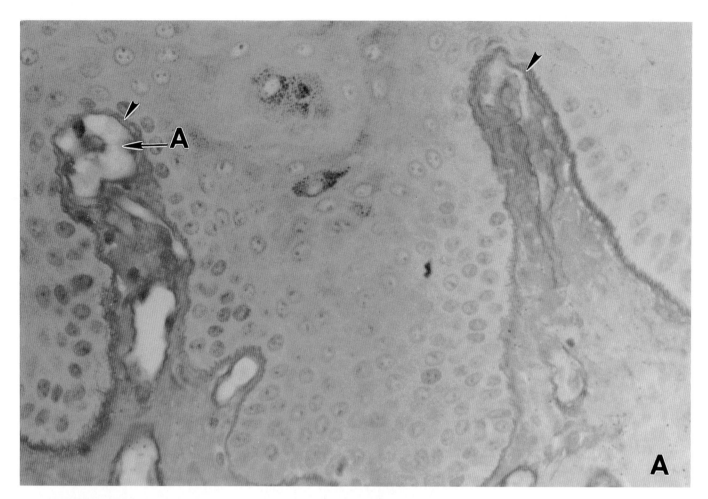

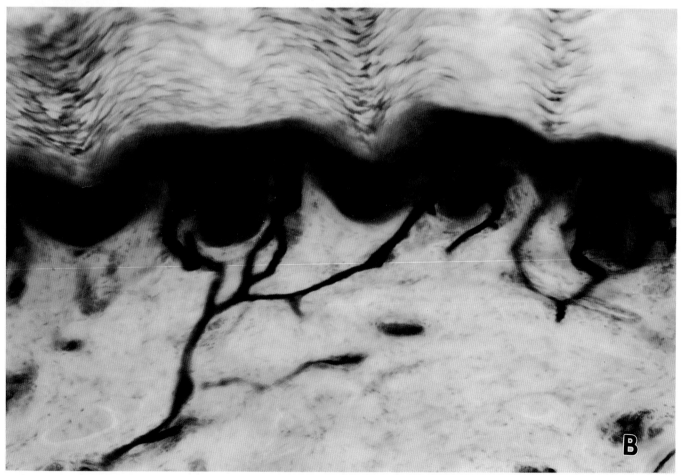

PLATE 81

CAPILLARY LOOPS

Aging

Capillary loops in the ball of the finger of the young are formed of two or three vessels in each epidermal ridge and follow the lines of the fingerprint. The vascular patterns alter with aging; there is multiplication of the loops from simple to complex ones. In elderly people, some capillary loops are lost and new ones arise from the interpapillary network.

A. SEM micrograph of a resin cast of the fine vasculature of the finger of an 85-year-old man shows a complex "thicket" pattern of capillary loops in the dermal ridges. OM 150x. Courtesy of Prof. A. Ikeda.

B. There are several types of loops in the finger of an 85-year-old man. The interpapillary capillary networks are particularly evident. Resin cast, SEM. OM 150x. Courtesy of Prof. A. Ikeda.

C. SEM micrograph of individual capillary loops in the finger of an 85-year-old man. There are simple loops on the right and multiple ones on the left. Resin cast. OM 700x. Courtesy of Prof. A. Ikeda.

D. Bunched capillary loops are evident in this SEM micrograph of a resin cast of the heel of an 85-year-old man. OM 300x. Courtesy of Prof. A. Ikeda.

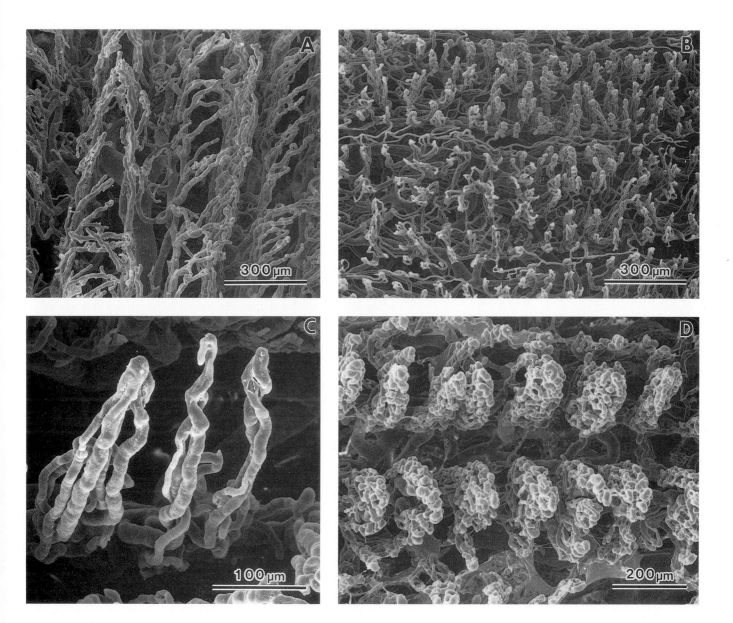

PLATE 82

CAPILLARIES

A. Capillary loop (C) with its ascending and descending segments in the papillary dermis of the chin of a middle-aged man. 2-μm plastic section. Verhoff's hematoxylin. OM 400x.

B. This longitudinal section of a capillary in the reticular dermis of a middle-aged man shows that the lumen is just large enough to allow the passage of red blood cells (R). The endothelial cells (arrowheads) of the capillaries have long, flattened nuclei. 2-μm plastic section. Regaud's hematoxylin. OM 1000x.

C. This vessel in the reticular dermis of the facial skin of a young woman shows the characteristically odd-shaped nuclei of endothelial cells (E). The lumen contains red blood cells and the vessel is surrounded by fibroblasts and mast cells (M). 2-μm plastic section. Azure–eosin stain. OM 630x.

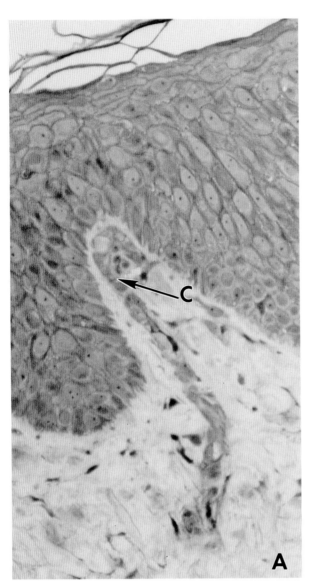

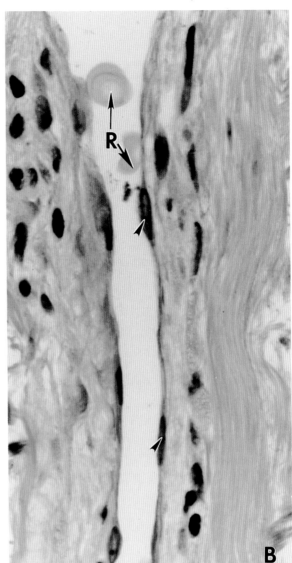

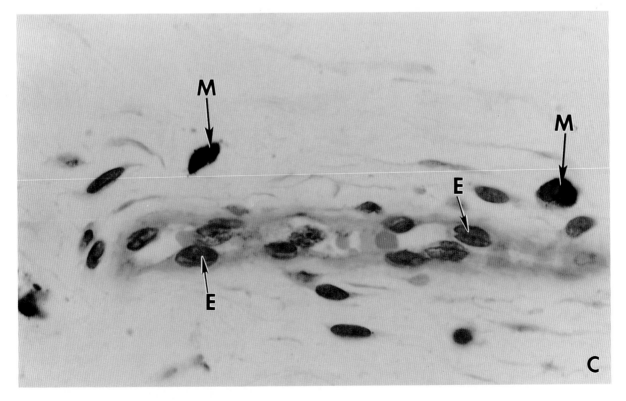

PLATE 83

VEINS and LYMPH VESSELS

A. Dermal veins (V) are always surrounded by a bed of fine collagenous fiber bundles that usually contain clusters of lymphocytes and other dermal cells. 2-μm plastic section. H and Lee. OM 250x.

B. Lymphatic vessels regulate tissue pressure and clear away effete cells, proteins, fluids, and degraded materials. Lymphatic vessels (L) have valves (arrow) that maintain one-way flow and prevent backflow. The thin endothelial lining of this lymphatic vessel sits directly on the connective tissue without a specialized bed of fine collagenous fibers. Compare this vessel with the nearby venule (V). Capillary (C). From the facial skin of a 65-year-old Black woman. 4-μm plastic section. Verhoff's elastic fiber technique. OM 250x.

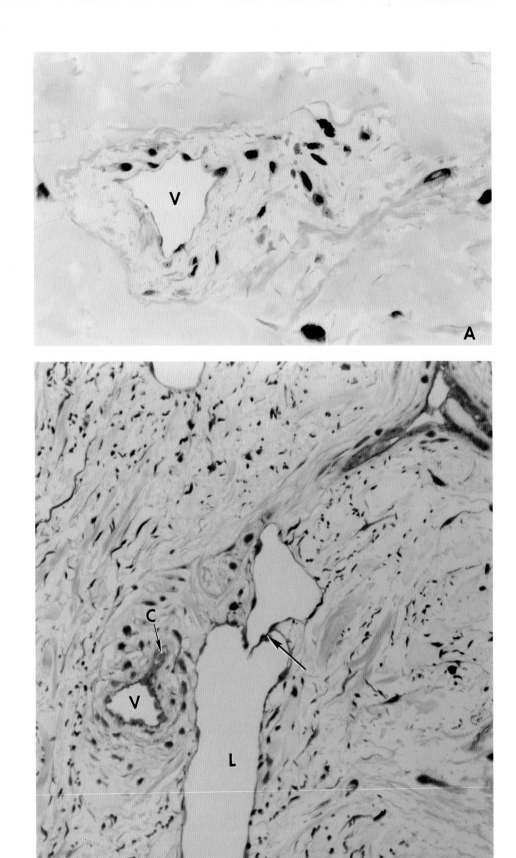

PLATE 84

LYMPHATIC VESSELS

Skin is very rich in lymphatic vessels. Lymphatic vessels do not show up well in routine sections and their study has been neglected. They are extremely important in transferring interstitial macromolecules and cells back to the circulation. Lymphatics can be visualized by injecting Berlin blue intradermally and photographing the spread of the dye in the lymphatic vessels that are visible at the surface. All of the figures were photographed at approximately 2x. Courtesy of Prof. D. Lubach.

A. Two small "initial" lymphatic drainage fields just under the dermal–epidermal junction of back skin, opening into a larger lymphatic channel (arrow) deeper in the papillary dermis, below the level of the venular plexus.

B. These two merging drainage fields are deeper in the papillary dermis (100 to 200 μm below the dermal–epidermal junction) than those shown in Figure A.

C. These lymphatic vessels, deeper still in the papillary dermis, have a slightly wider lumen and form wider meshes than those in Figures A and B.

D. High magnification of the lymphatic channels shown in Figure C.

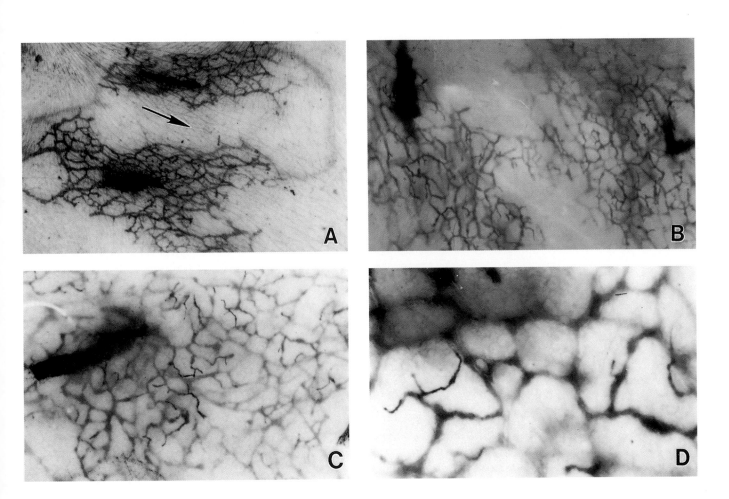

PLATE 85

ARTERIES

Aging Changes

A. The basement membranes (BM) of small arteries (A) and an arteriole (At) from the facial skin of a 26-year-old man are PAS-reactive, indicating that they contain a mixture of proteoglycans and other PAS-reactive substances. The sarcolemma (sa) of the muscle cells is also PAS-reactive. 4-μm plastic section. PAS. OM 630x.

B. The architecture of these small arterioles from the facial skin of a 70-year-old man is greatly altered by aging and sun exposure. Degenerative changes are obvious and are certain to hamper normal function. 4-μm plastic section. PAS. OM 630x.

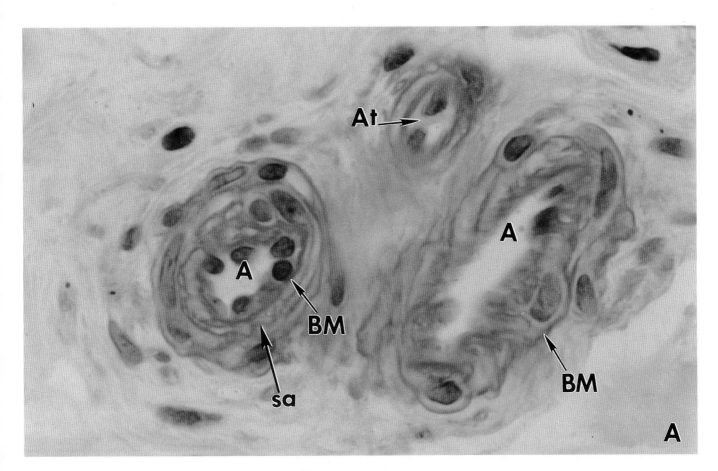

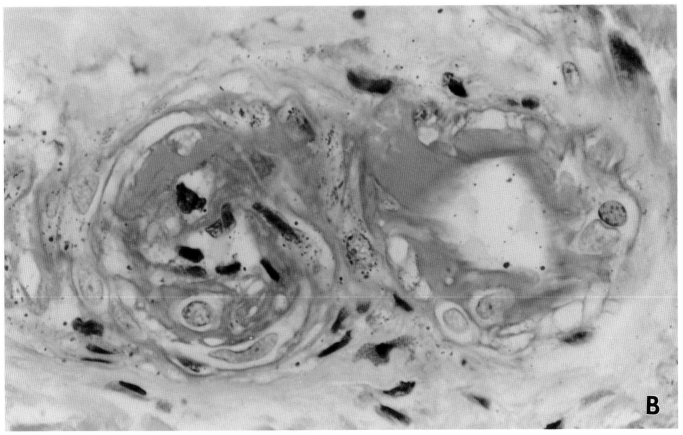

PLATE 86

ARTERIES

A. An artery (A) from the lip of a 20-year-old man. Most of the elastic fibers in the tunica elastica interna are oriented longitudinally. The tunica elastica interna of arteries is an elastic fiber compartment, the skeleton of the arteries. Veins (V) lack an internal elastic membrane. The few elastic fibers are found primarily in the adventitia. 60-μm frozen section. Roman's AOV elastic fiber technique. OM 120x.

B. In this muscular artery from the finger of a 20-year-old woman, the tunica elastica interna (arrow) shows the longitudinally oriented elastic fibers. The muscle cells are surrounded by very fine elastic fibers that stain black and purple. 30-μm frozen section. Weigert's elastic fiber technique. OM 200x.

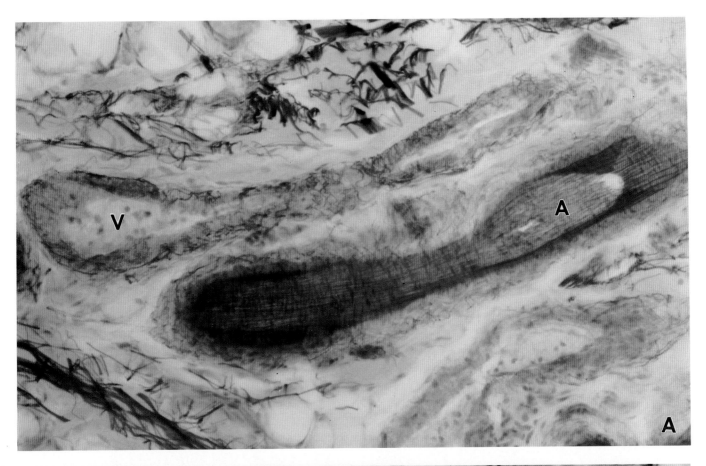

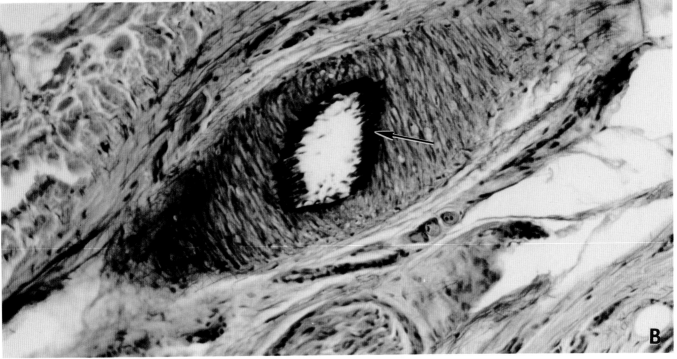

PLATE 87

TRIAD

Artery, Vein, and Nerve

This "triad" from the facial skin of a 35-year-old man consists of an artery (A), a vein (V), and a nerve (N). The individual, longitudinally oriented elastic fibers of the tunica elastica interna (E) identify this vessel as an artery. The accompanying collapsed vein has only a few smooth muscle cells in its wall and very few elastic fibers. 4-μm plastic section. Verhoff's elastic fiber technique. OM 630x.

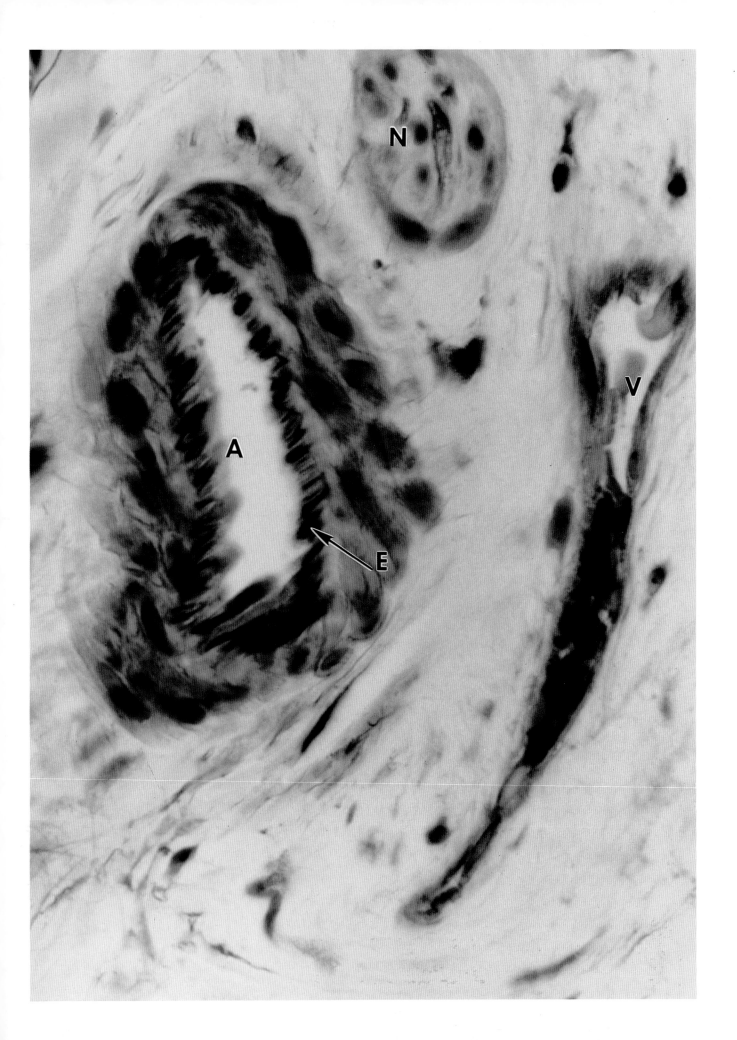

PLATE 88

ARTERIOVENOUS ANASTOMOSES

In 1628 Harvey described the circulation of blood from arteries to veins, and Malpighi in 1661 showed that blood passes from arteries to veins by way of capillaries. In 1707 Lealis observed that blood in the spermatic artery passes directly into the spermatic vein. Subsequently, Suquet in 1862 and Hoyer in 1873 demonstrated the existence of many shunts that directly connect arterioles to venules. These shunts, or arteriovenous anastomoses, form a specialized vascular unit called the glomus body in the hands and feet. These structures, also sometimes referred to as Suquet-Hoyer anastomoses, are particularly well developed in the terminal phalanges of the digits, the tip of the nose, the lips, and the auricular pavilion. They aid in the regulation of blood flow.

A. In the skin of the hands and feet, blood can go directly from arterioles to venules through the arteriovenous anastomoses or glomuses. The one shown here from the finger of a 36-year-old man is a thick-walled, muscular artery with a narrow lumen. Like all smooth muscle cells, the muscle cells in the glomus have a PAS-reactive sarcolemma and glycogen granules in the sarcoplasm. 4-μm plastic section. PAS counterstained with hematoxylin. OM 250x.

B. The primary role of the glomus is temperature regulation; in response to lower temperatures, the capillaries shut down. In this section of finger skin of a 34-year-old woman, the glomus (G) has a thick, muscular coat. Smooth muscle cells of the wall are surrounded by fine reticulin fibers. Large nerves (N) are always associated with the glomus. 4-μm plastic section. Gridley's reticulin fiber technique. OM 160x.

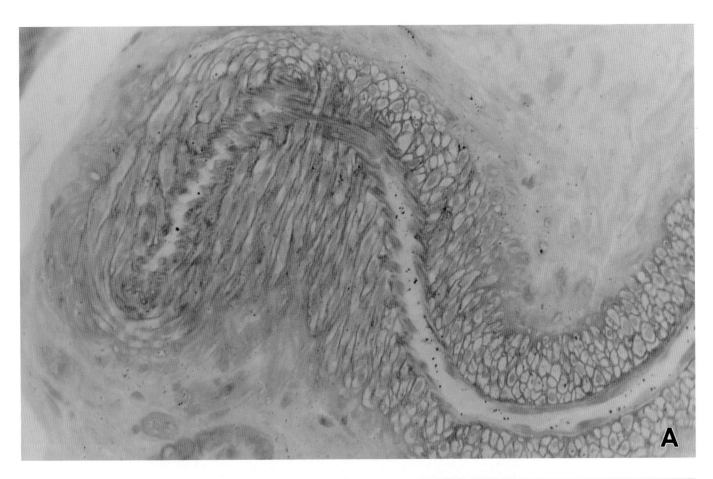

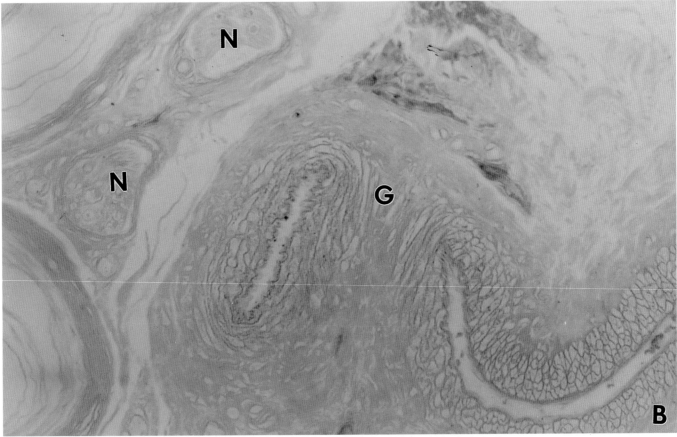

PLATE 89

ARTERY

Innervation

A. Depending on their location in the body, arteries can have a rich or a sparse innervation. Nerves mediate constriction and dilation of arteries, thus regulating blood flow, which in turn regulates body temperature. This artery, near the corpus cavernosum in the clitoris of a 20-year-old woman, is cloaked in a dense net of acetylcholinesterase-reactive nerves. The tumescence and detumescence of the genitalia are determined by blood flow. 60-μm frozen section. Koelle's acetylcholinesterase technique. OM 100x.

B. This artery (A) from the chin of a 21-year-old man contains only a few acetylcholinesterase-reactive nerves between the smooth muscle cells of the tunica adventitia. Vein (V). 60-μm frozen section. Koelle's acetylcholinesterase technique. OM 160x.

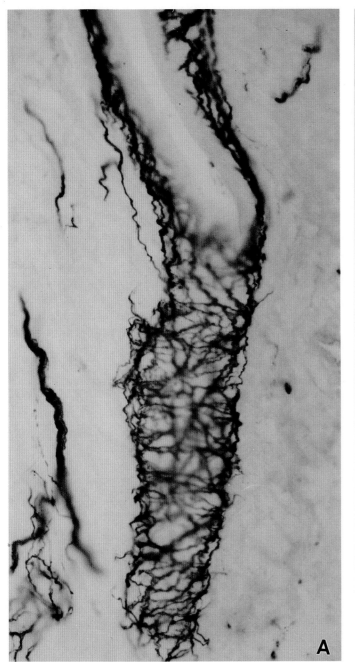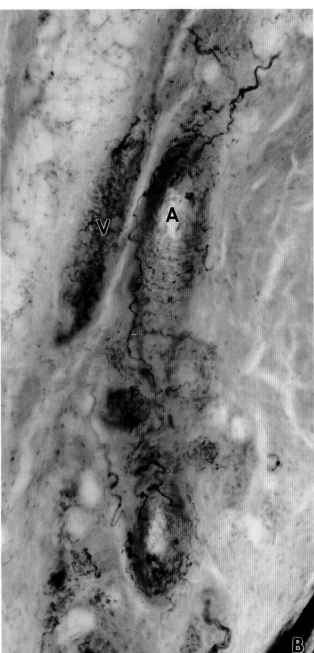

PLATE 90

BLOOD VESSEL

TEM micrograph of a blood vessel from the face of a young Black woman. Endothelial cells (E) surround the lumen of the vessel. The thick, homogeneous arterial basement membrane encloses collagen and smooth muscle cells, the pericytes (P). In contrast, the basement membrane of a venule is characterized by a laminated appearance, with dense layers of collagen alternating with the homogeneous component of the basement membrane. The individual vessels of the microcirculatory system have the same basic structure, and the small vessels are difficult to identify. A veil cell (V) near the vessel maintains the tone of the vessel wall. The arrows indicate the cytoplasmic extensions ("wings") of the veil cell that surround the vessel. A binucleated fibroblast (F) and collagenous bundles (C) are seen in the surrounding dermis. OM 3900x.

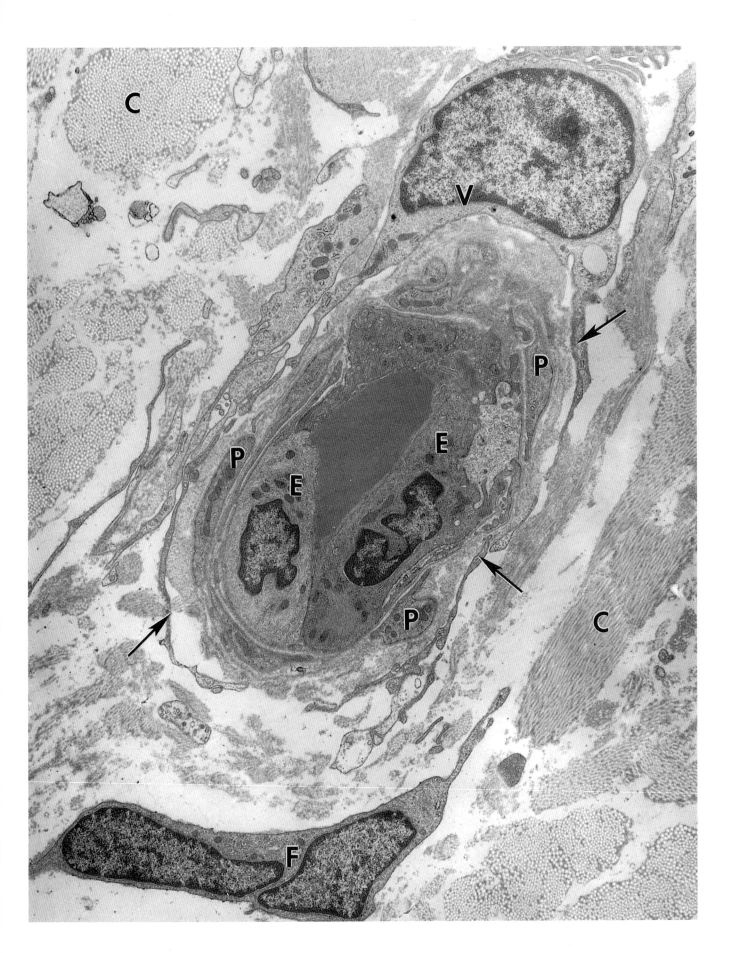

Skin Sensory Mechanisms

The skin, the largest sense organ of the body, is the interface between the organism and its environment. It must ensure that the organism is able to perceive all environmental changes, both pleasurable ones and those that threaten its existence. Tactile receptors are spread over the roughly two square meters of the body surface, whereas all of the other major sensory organs are crowded into the head. Cutaneous nerves contain sensory and sympathetic (autonomic) nerve fibers. The sympathetic motor fibers, mixed with the sensory fibers in the dermis, eventually send branches to the sweat glands, blood vessels, and arrectores pilorum muscles. The sensory fibers and their specialized corpuscular end organs are receptors for touch, pain, temperature, itch, and physical and chemical stimuli. A large portion of the human sensory cortex receives sensory messages from the skin of the face and the hands, areas that are especially well supplied with receptor organs.

PLATE 91

INTRAEPIDERMAL NERVES

The existence of intraepidermal nerves in human skin has been debated in the past. New techniques, including monoclonal antibodies to nerve components, have unequivocally demonstrated their presence everywhere. Intraepidermal nerves appear to be both myelinated and nonmyelinated. Winkelmann's nerve technique demonstrates myelinated nerves, and Koelle's acetylcholinesterase technique shows nonmyelinated nerves.

A. Rich network of acetylcholinesterase-reactive nerves under an epidermal ridge of the lip of a 21-year-old man. Some of these nerves appear to penetrate the epidermis (Ep) for a short distance (arrows). 20-μm frozen section. Koelle's acetylcholinesterase technique. OM 200x.

B. Intraepidermal nerves are numerous in fetal skin. These myelinated nerves (arrows), in the labia minora of an 8-month fetus, appear to penetrate the epidermis (Ep). 30-μm frozen section. Winkelmann's nerve technique. OM 200x.

C. Intraepidermal nerves are well developed in the rhinarium of moles, opossums, and tree shrews. Adult human beings have only vestiges of these nerves. However, inside the choanae of the internal nares, where there are no hairs, the thick epidermis has numerous intraepidermal nerves (arrows), as in the nose of this 67-year-old man. 20-μm frozen section. Winkelmann's nerve technique. OM 520x.

D. An intraepidermal nerve, from the internal nares of a 67-year-old man, rises through the stratum granulosum (arrow). The exoplasm of intraepidermal nerves may grow at a rate that keeps pace with the shedding of the corneocytes. 20-μm frozen section. Winkelmann's nerve technique. OM 520x.

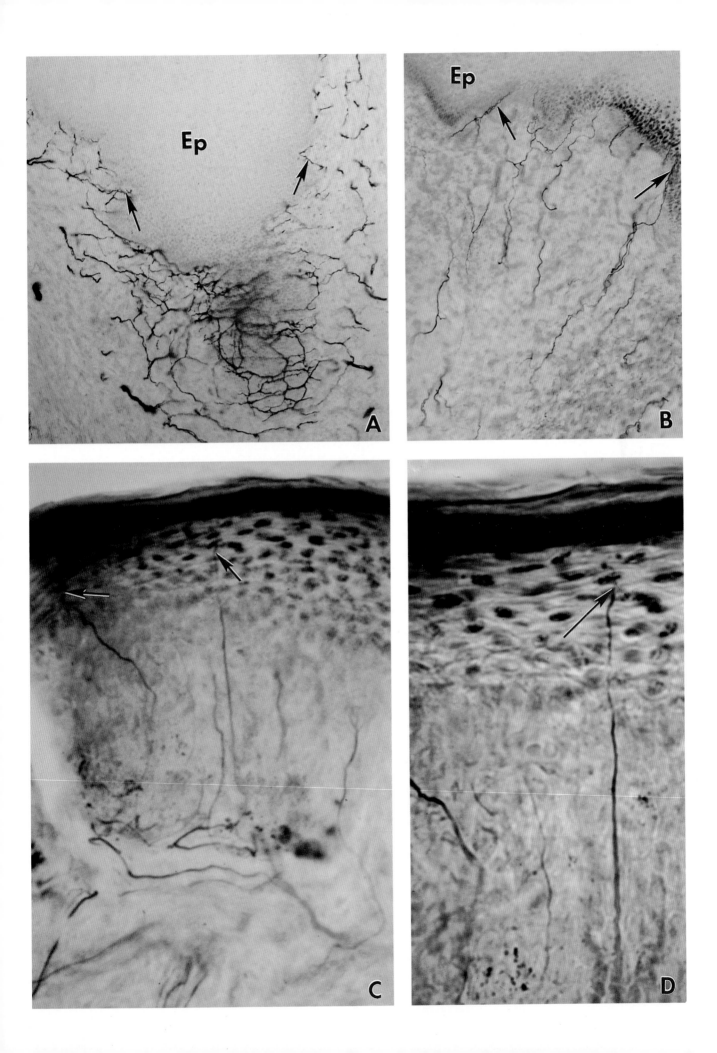

PLATE 92

NERVE

Face

The face is innervated by cutaneous branches of the trigeminal nerve. Free nerve endings in the papillary dermis are always accompanied by Schwann cells and a basal lamina.

TEM micrograph of the concentric myelin (My) layers around a nerve (N) from the face of a Black woman; the nucleus (Nu) of a Schwann cell is above the nerve. Note also the nonmyelinated nerve (NN) fibers surrounded by Schwann cells (arrow). Basal lamina (BL). Collagen (C). OM 32,000x.

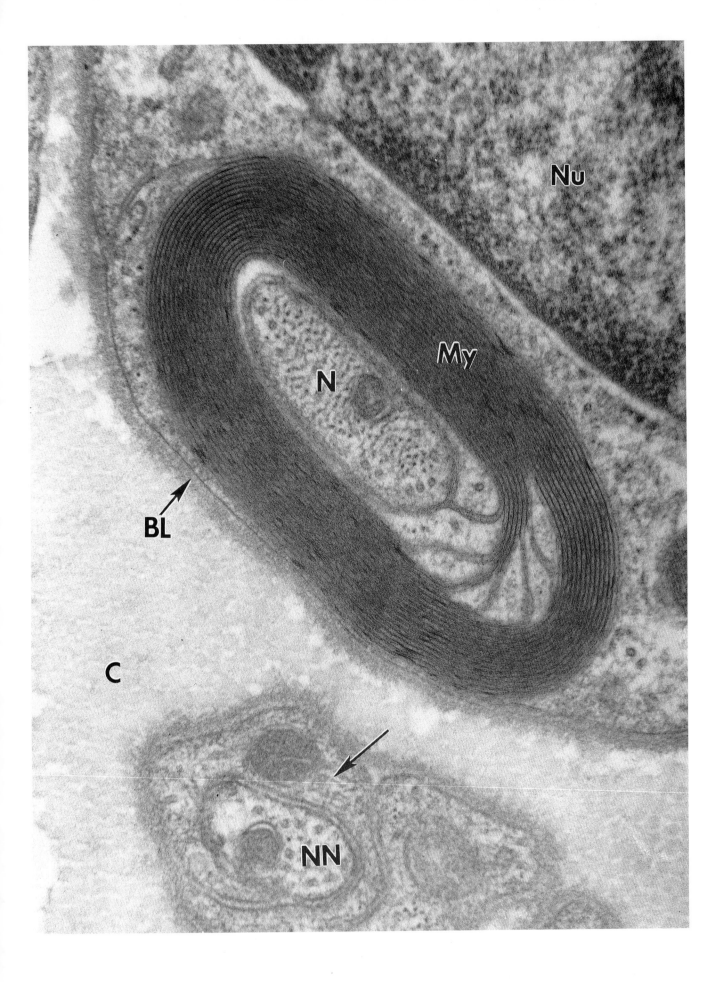

PLATE 93

SENSORY NERVES

Free nerve endings—the most widespread and the most important sensory receptors—and the end organs function together. All sensory receptor end organs, also known as corpuscles, are built on a similar structural plan; they contain both neural and nonneural components. The end organs include mucocutaneous end organs, Meissner corpuscles, and pacinian corpuscles. Except for those of the Meissner corpuscle, the connective tissue capsules are a continuation of the perineurium. The neural elements of all end organs consist of both nonmyelinated and myelinated nerves. The density and types of receptors vary by region.

A. Intraepidermal nonmyelinated nerves (arrows) in the epidermis (Ep) of the labia minora of a 12-year-old girl. Intraepidermal nerves are more common in fetal skin and in healing wounds. The large brown bodies are genital corpuscles (G) or mucocutaneous end organs. 30-μm frozen section. Koelle's acetylcholinesterase technique. OM 250x.

B. A penicillate free nerve ending of Cauna (arrows), from the nose of a 20-year-old man, is one of many in this region. To visualize the penicillate, branching arrangement, serial sections must be cut and a model reconstructed. 40-μm frozen section. Winkelmann's silver impregnation method. OM 160x.

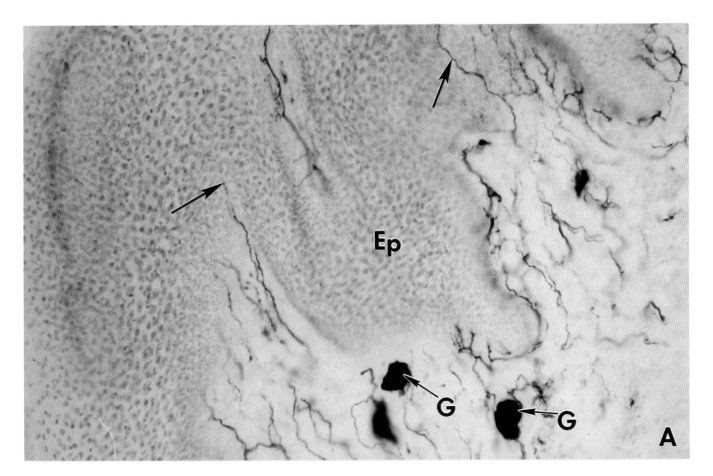

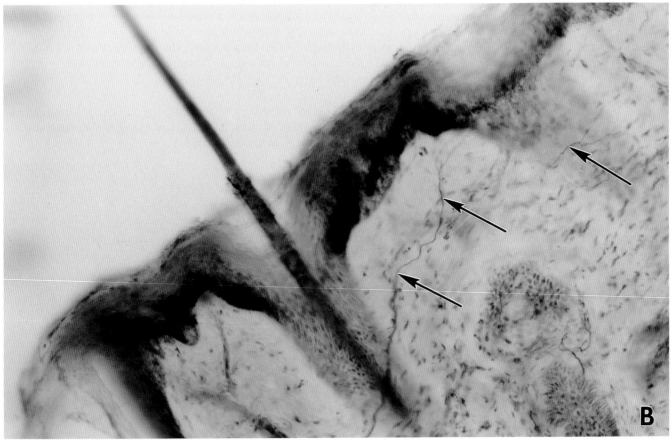

PLATE 94

SENSORY NERVES
Genitalia

Encapsulated end organs are numerous in such glabrous areas as the lips, the labia, the glans penis, and the areolae of women's breasts. There is a gradual waning of hair follicles and an increase in mucocutaneous end organs in transitional areas from cutaneous to mucous surfaces.

A. Clitoris (C) and corpora cavernosa (CC) of an 18-year-old woman. There are many genital corpuscles (G) and nonmyelinated nerves throughout the tissue. 20-μm frozen section. Koelle's acetylcholinesterase technique. OM 100x.

B. The clitoris abounds in myelinated nerves (arrows) and genital corpuscles (G). From an 18-year-old woman. 30-μm frozen section. Winkelmann's silver impregnation method. OM 125x.

C. The vagina is richly supplied with fine subepidermal nonmyelinated nerves that almost reach the mucosa. From a 12-year-old girl. 20-μm frozen section. Koelle's acetylcholinesterase technique. OM 125x.

D. Many nerves (arrows) and genital corpuscles (G) in the glans penis of a 20-year-old man. 30-μm frozen section. Winkelmann's silver impregnation method. OM 125x.

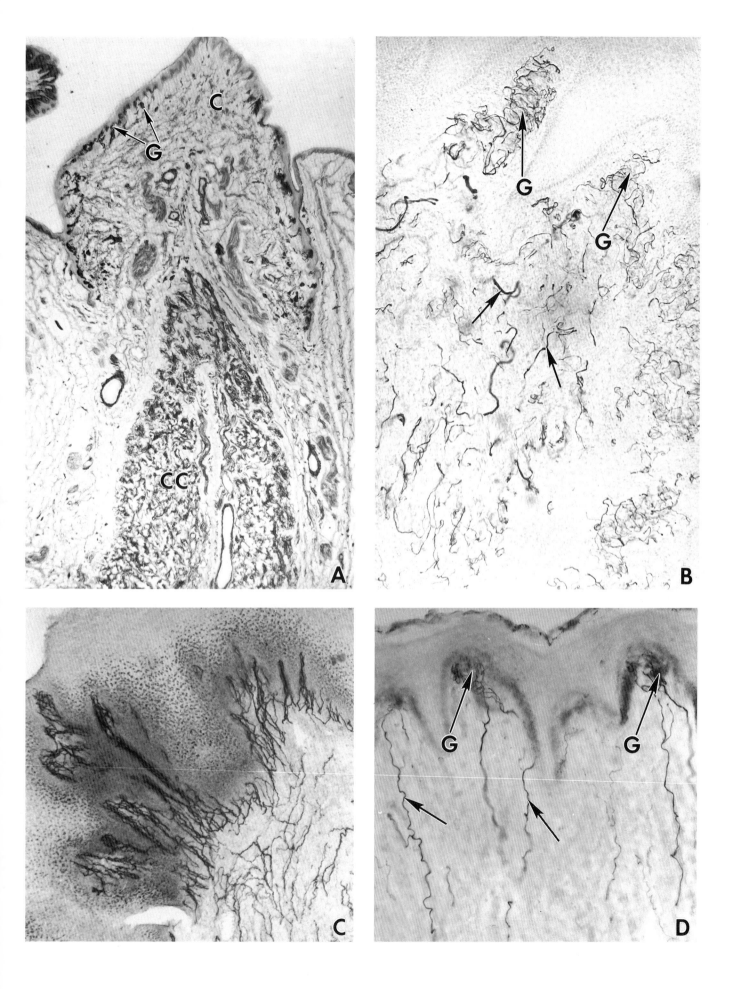

PLATE 95

GENITAL CORPUSCLES

A. Acetylcholinesterase-reactive nerves (arrows) and genital corpuscles (G) in the labia minora of a 12-year-old girl. The connective tissue elements of all encapsulated and semiencapsulated end organs, as well as many nonmyelinated nerves, are equally reactive for acetylcholinesterase. 20μm frozen section. Koelle's acetylcholinesterase technique. OM 200x.

B. Genital corpuscles (G) and myelinated nerves (arrow) in the labia minora of a 19-year-old woman. 20-μm frozen section. Winkelmann's silver impregnation method. OM 200x.

C. The genital corpuscles (G) in the glans penis of an 18-year-old man, like those in female external genitalia, are strongly reactive for acetylcholinesterase. Note the intraepidermal nerves (arrow). 15-μm frozen section. Koelle's acetylcholinesterase technique. OM 200x.

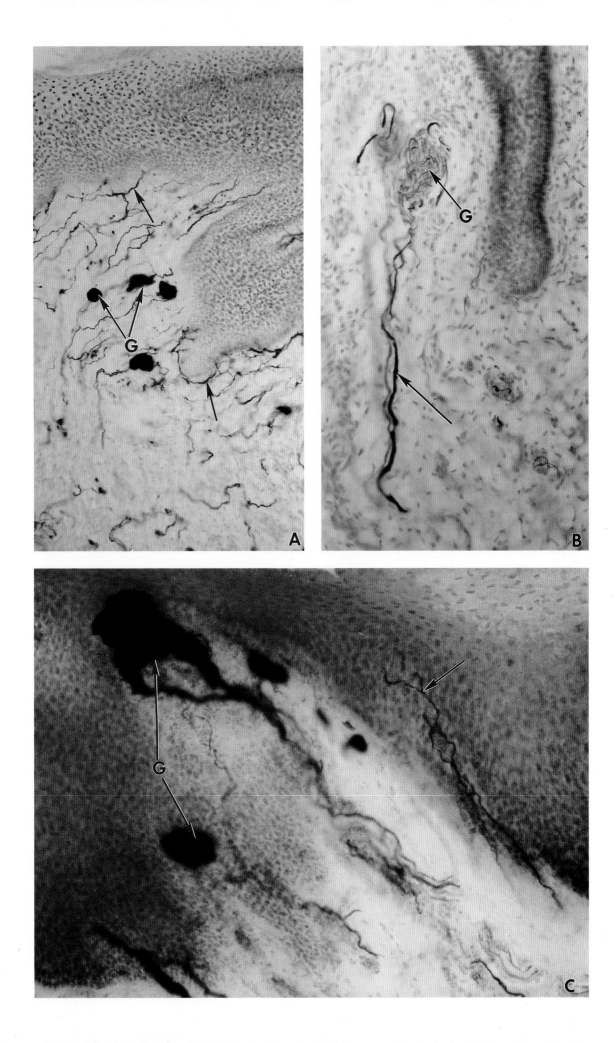

PLATE 96

MUCOCUTANEOUS
END ORGANS

A. Genital corpuscle (G) in the glans penis of an 18-year-old man; genital corpuscles are similar in men and women. In men the nerves are very fine, and the corpuscles are nearly always close to the epidermis and are rarely found deep in the connective tissue. 30-μm frozen section. Winkelmann's silver impregnation method. OM 160x.

B. Although mucocutaneous end organs are mainly distributed in glabrous skin, they can also be found throughout the skin of the face, where they are known as Krause's end bulbs. This corpuscle is from an ala of the nose of an old man. 30-μm frozen section. Winkelmann's silver impregnation method. OM 250x.

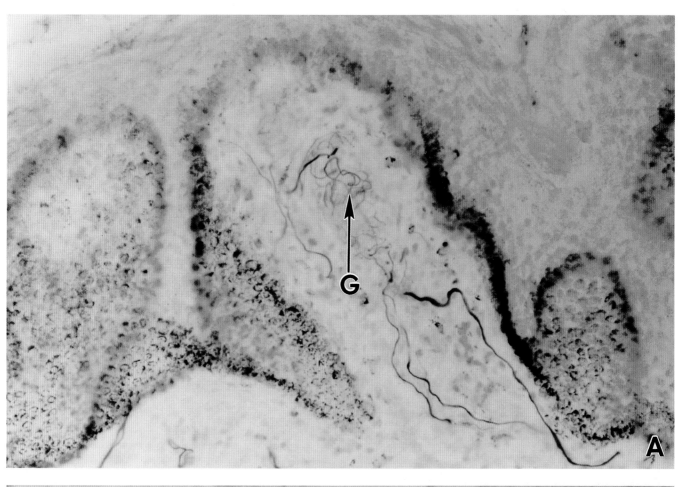

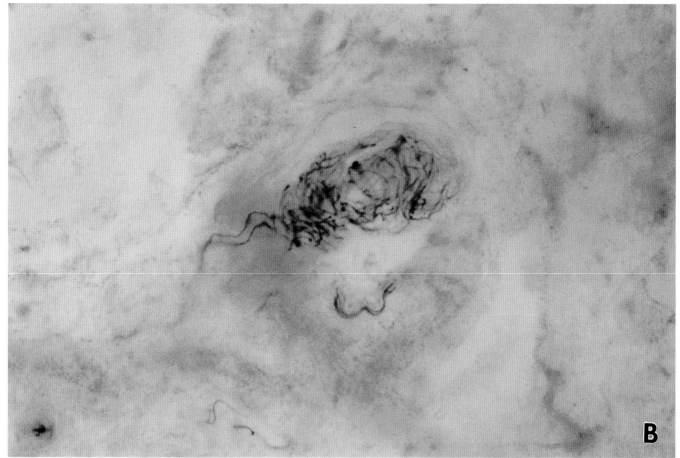

PLATE 97

MUCOCUTANEOUS END ORGANS

A. Mucocutaneous end organs (M) and intraepidermal nerves (arrows) in the lip of an 8-month fetus. 20-μm frozen section. Koelle's acetylcholinesterase technique. OM 160x.

B. Mucocutaneous end organs (M) and myelinated nerves (arrows) in the upper lip of a 63-year-old man. 20-μm frozen section. Winkelmann's silver impregnation method. OM 100x.

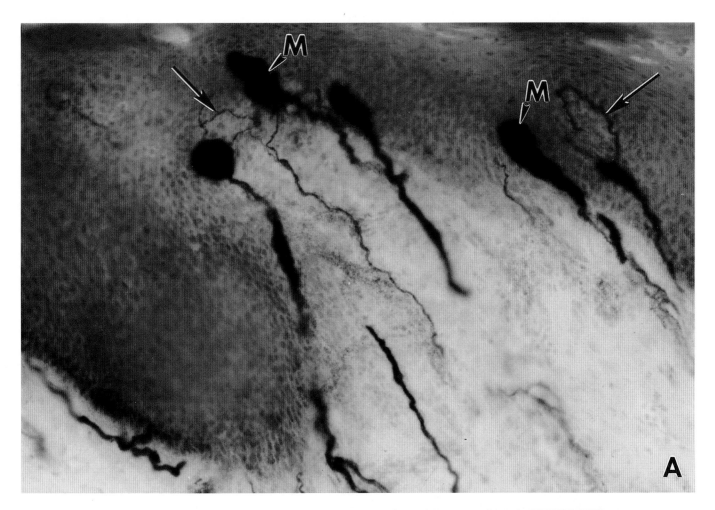

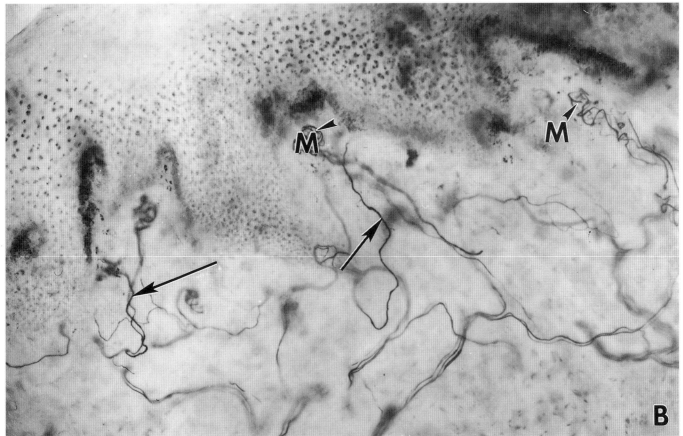

PLATE 98

MEISSNER CORPUSCLES

The hands and feet of human beings are richly supplied with the special sensory organs, Meissner corpuscles. These ellipsoid receptors are located just under the epidermis. The mucocutaneous end organs on the lips, the genital corpuscles, and the Meissner corpuscles each consist of tightly wound, capsule-enclosed balls of a single, branching nerve or group of nerves.

A. Myelinated axons enter the base of the Meissner corpuscle (M) and terminate in endings that are surrounded by specialized Schwann cells, the laminar cells (arrow). Connective tissue cells, collagenous fibers, and elastic fibers surround the nerve fibers and provide support. Blood vessel (bv). From the finger of a 34-year-old woman. 2-μm plastic section. H and Lee. OM 500x.

B. The horizontal alignment (arrow) and the intense magenta staining of the laminar cells of a Meissner corpuscle (M) in the finger of a 36-year-old man. Note the intraepidermal mast cell (Ma), a rarity. 2-μm plastic section. Giemsa stain. OM 630x.

C. This Meissner corpuscle (M) from the finger of a 34-year-old woman shows the strong PAS reactivity of its extracellular elements and of the basement membrane (BM) under the epidermis. 4-μm plastic section. PAS. OM 630x.

D. The laminar cells in this Meissner corpuscle (M) in the finger of a 36-year-old man are outlined with reticulin fibers. Similar reticulin fibers accompany the epidermal basement membrane (BM). 4-μm plastic section. Gridley's reticulin fiber technique. OM 630x.

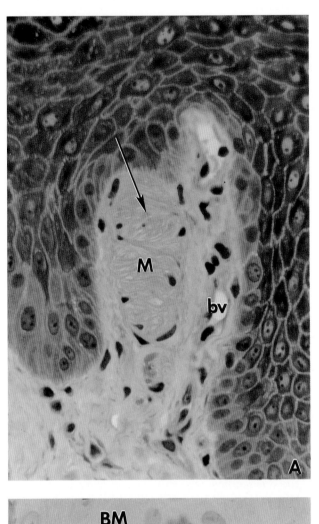

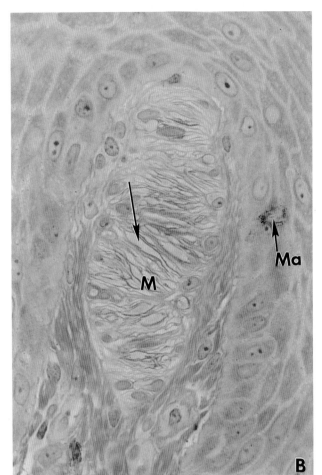

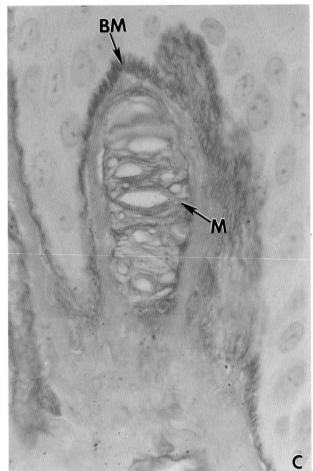

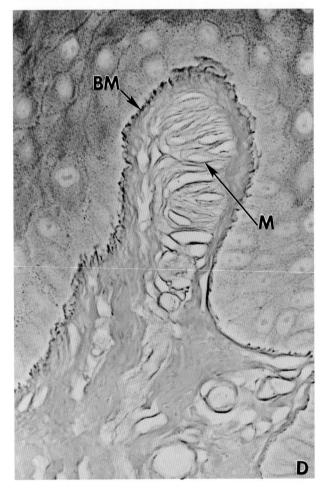

PLATE 99

MEISSNER/PACINIAN CORPUSCLES

A. Cocoon-like Meissner corpuscle (M) slung from the epidermis by silk-like elastic fibers in the finger skin of a 6-year-old girl. There are no elastic fibers inside the corpuscles. 30-μm frozen section. Roman's AOV elastic fiber technique. OM 160x.

B. A pacinian corpuscle (PC), the largest and most highly structured of all corpuscles, is also held in place by spiderweb-like elastic fibers. Note that fine elastic fibers also penetrate the capsule and accompany the concentric collagenous fiber laminae. From the finger of a young man. 20-μm frozen section. Weigert's elastic fiber technique. OM 160x.

C. Meissner corpuscles (M) and nerves (arrows) in the finger of a 6-year-old girl are strongly acetylcholinesterase-reactive. The neural elements and the surrounding connective tissue cells are reactive for both acetylcholinesterase and butyrylcholinesterase, which suggests that this enzyme is a nonspecific esterase. Note the stratum lucidum (L) and stratum corneum (C) in the thick epidermis. Koelle's acetylcholinesterase technique. OM 160x.

D. Coiled axon of a Meissner corpuscle (M) from the finger skin of a 30-year-old man. 30-μm frozen section. Winkelmann's silver impregnation method. OM 160x.

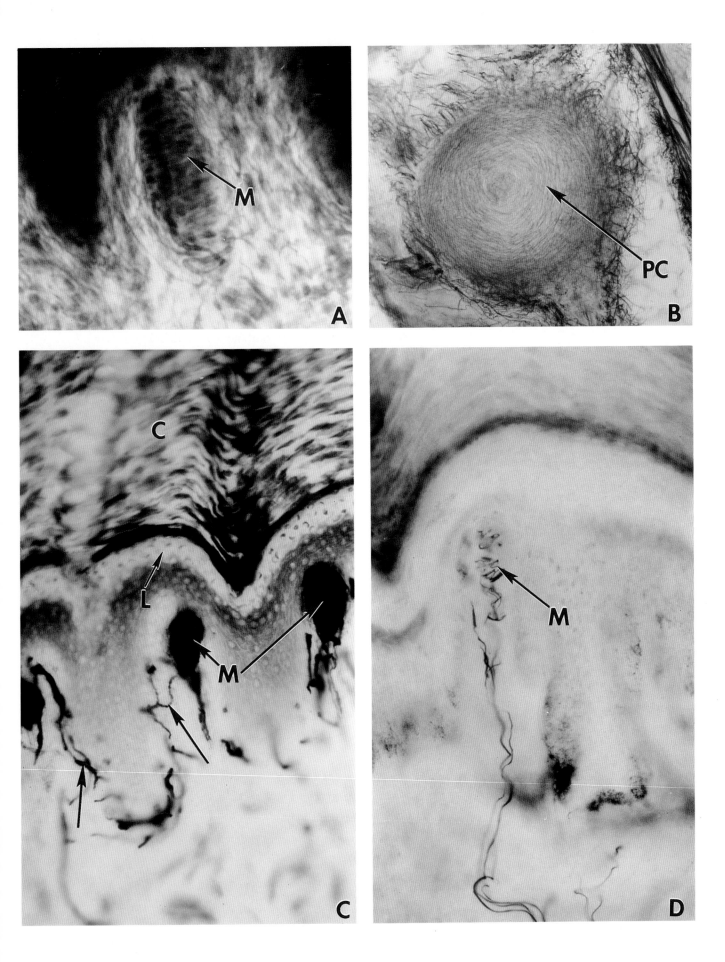

PLATE 100

MEISSNER/PACINIAN CORPUSCLES

A, B, C, and D. Meissner corpuscles cut in different planes to show the twisting loops of the long, branching nerve in each. Myelinated axons enter the base of the capsule and twist repeatedly. 20-μm frozen section. Winkelmann's nerve technique. OM 160x.

E. Transverse section through two pacinian corpuscles (P), the largest sensory receptors in the body. Depending on their location, pacinian corpuscles vary from 0.2 to 1 mm in diameter. Note the central body (C), intracapsular blood vessels (bv), and large accompanying nerves (N) in the finger skin of a 34-year-old woman. 2-μm plastic section. Roman's AOV elastic fiber technique. OM 160x.

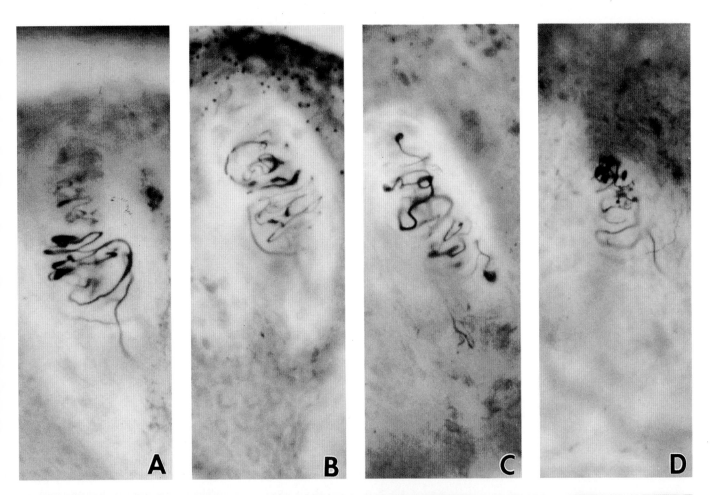

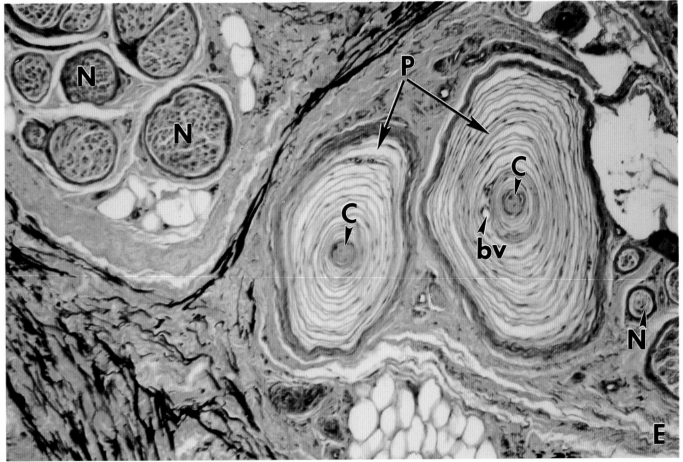

PLATE 101

PACINIAN CORPUSCLES

Pacinian corpuscles, considered to be deep pressure receptors that respond to vibrational stimuli, are numerous in the fingers, clitoris, mesenteries, and pancreas. Each corpuscle has a central body surrounded by a capsule that is shaped like an onion. Pacinian corpuscles are distinguished by the lamellar wrappings of their capsule. The capsule consists of an outer zone containing concentric layers of cells and fibrous connective tissue; a middle zone composed of collagenous fibers, elastic fibers, and fibroblasts; and an inner zone made up of Schwann cells. The lamellated structure functions as a mechanical filter that restricts the range of response.

A. Longitudinal and transverse cuts through the central body or inner core (C) of pacinian corpuscles from the hand of a 6-year-old girl. The concentric collagenous sheets also contain very fine elastic fibers. 30-μm frozen section. Reichert's elastic fiber technique. OM 160x.

B. The nerves (N) and inner core (C) of this transversely cut pacinian corpuscle are reactive for acetylcholinesterase; the concentric connective tissue laminae that surround it are not. 20-μm frozen section. Koelle's acetylcholinesterase technique. OM 160x.

C. The longitudinally cut inner core (C) of a pacinian corpuscle, and the nerves that surround it, are reactive for acetylcholinesterase. The blood vessels (bv) are surrounded by many nerves. From the hand of a 6-year-old girl. 20-μm frozen section. Koelle's acetylcholinesterase technique. OM 160x.

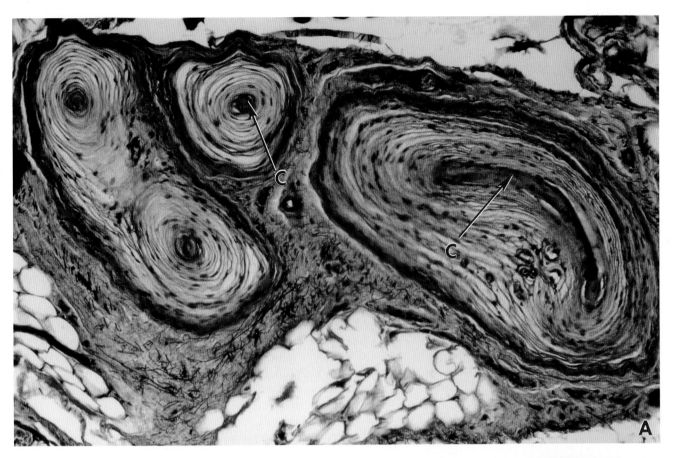

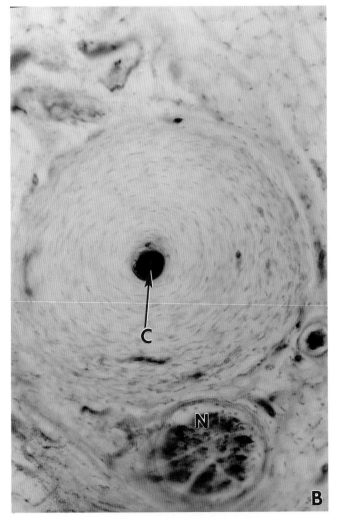

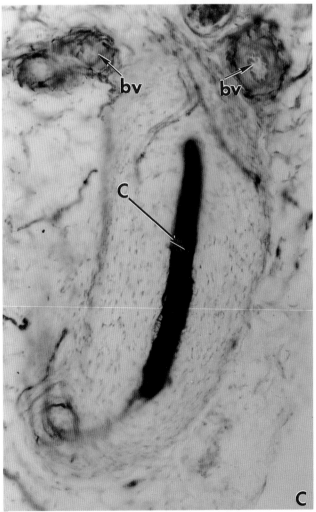

PLATE 102

NERVES
Hair Follicle

Man and whales are the only mammals with no vibrissae, but in man, this deficiency is compensated by a generous innervation of all hair follicles. Hair follicle nerve end organs are the most widespread sensory receptor organs; regardless of where the follicles are found, the structural plan of their end organs is similar.

Diagram of a vellus follicle surrounded by myelinated nerves. Every follicle is surrounded by nerve fibers from the base of the bulb to its junction with the epidermis. The patterns of nerves, more precise around vellus than larger follicles, are so well organized that they can be referred to as follicle end organs. The axons in hair follicle end organs, like those in genital and Meissner corpuscles, are reactive for acetylcholinesterases.

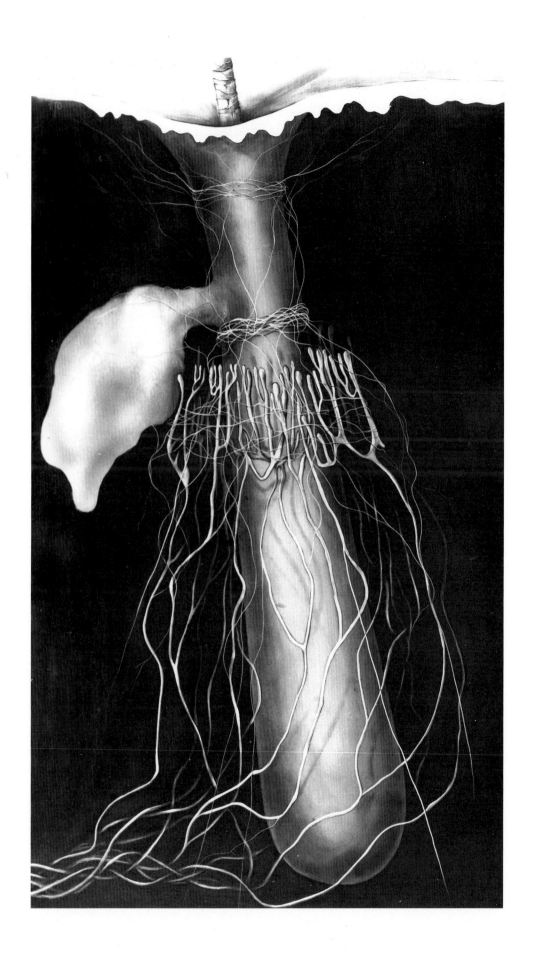

PLATE 103

NERVES
Hair Follicle

A. Many acetylcholinesterase-reactive nerves (arrows) in a transverse section of a vellus hair follicle in the labia minora of a 12-year-old girl. Although the follicles of fetal lanugo hair normally drop out of the labia minora before birth, some hair follicles can remain there throughout postnatal life. Note the hair (H) and external root sheath (E). 20-μm frozen section. Koelle's acetylcholinesterase technique. OM 100x.

B. Lanugo hair (H) follicle nerve end organ in the labia minora of an 8-month fetus showing both horizontally and longitudinally oriented myelinated nerves (arrows). External root sheath (E). 20-μm frozen section. Winkelmann's nerve technique. OM 100x.

C. A transverse cut through a lanugo follicle in the fetal labia minora shows that the myelinated nerves form a nerve "stockade" (arrow) around the follicle. Lanugo hair (H). Inner root sheath (IR). Sebaceous glands (sb). Myelinated nerve trunk (N). 20-μm frozen section. Winkelmann's nerve technique. OM 100x.

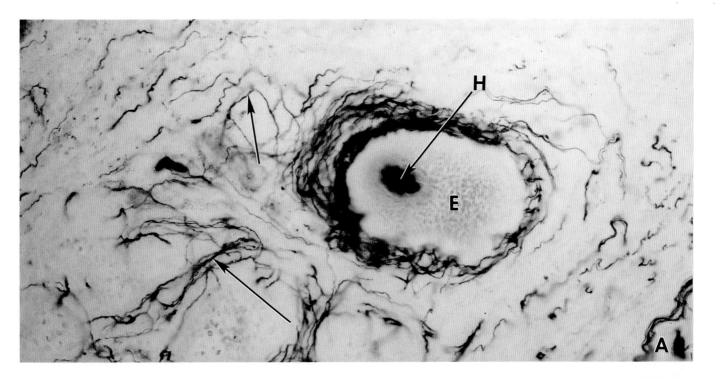

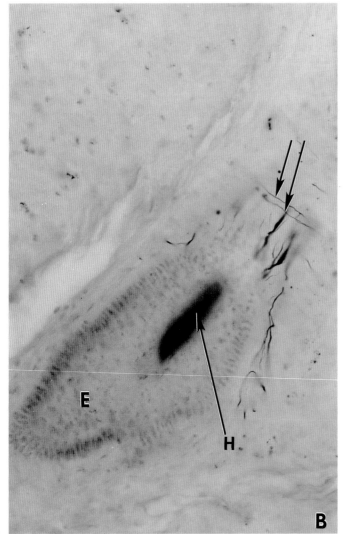

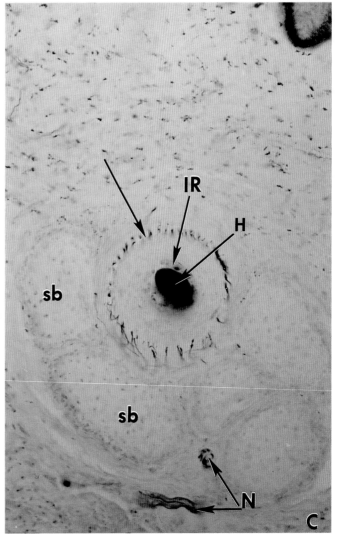

PLATE 104

NERVES

Hair Follicle

A. Myelinated nerves around an intermediate hair (hr) follicle from the nose of a 69-year-old man; this is the typical appearance of nerve end organs around the follicles of intermediate and terminal hairs. 15μm frozen section. Winkelmann's nerve technique. OM 160x.

B. Myelinated nerves around a vellus hair (hr) follicle in the earlobe of a 69-year-old man. 30-μm frozen section. Winkelmann's nerve technique. OM 160x.

C. Nerve "stockade" around a vellus hair (hr) follicle in the ear of a 69-year-old man. 30-μm frozen section. Winkelmann's nerve technique. OM 400x.

D. Details of some of the palisade nerve endings around a hair (hr) follicle from the same section as in Figure C. 30-μm frozen section. Winkelmann's nerve technique. OM 400x.

E. The myelinated nerves around the follicles of terminal hairs (hr) from the scalp of a 20-year-old man do not appear to be as well organized as those around vellus hair follicles. 30-μm frozen section. Winkelmann's nerve technique. OM 400x.

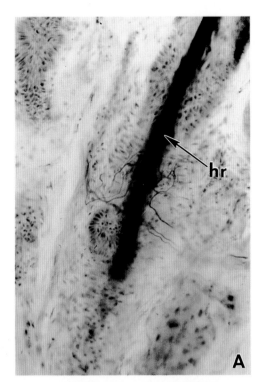

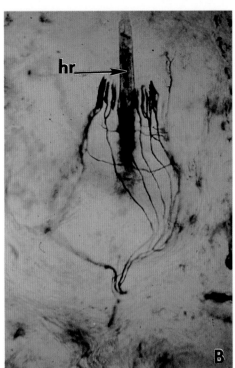

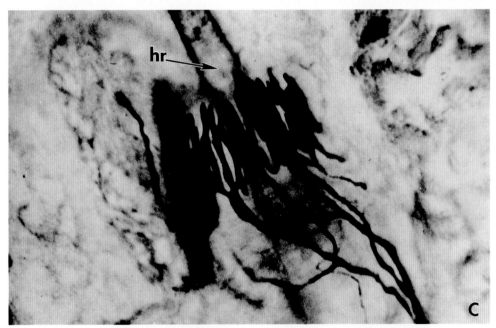

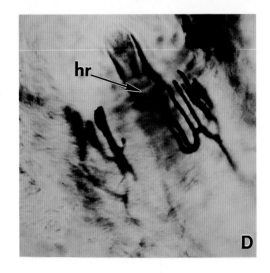

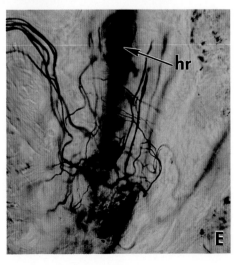

PLATE 105

NERVES

Hair Follicle

A. Every hair follicle at the tip of the nose of a 20-year-old man is equipped with a conspicuously acetylcholinesterase-reactive nerve end organ (arrows) and nerves. 30-μm frozen section. Koelle's acetylcholinesterase technique. OM 100x.

B. Acetylcholinesterase-reactive connective tissue capsule (arrow) around a vellus hair follicle from the nose of a 20-year-old man. 30-μm frozen section. Koelle's acetylcholinesterase technique. OM 100x.

C. This tangle of nerves around the canal (C) of a sebaceous follicle (sb) from the nose of a 20-year-old man is very likely a Haarscheibe, also called a tactile disk. Note the nerve end organ (arrow) around the vellus hair follicle. 30-μm frozen section. Koelle's acetylcholinesterase technique. OM 125x.

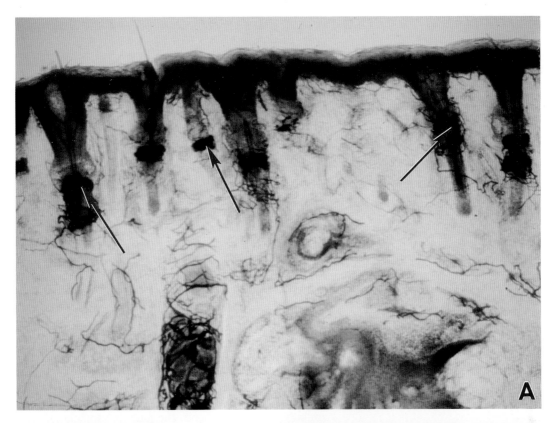

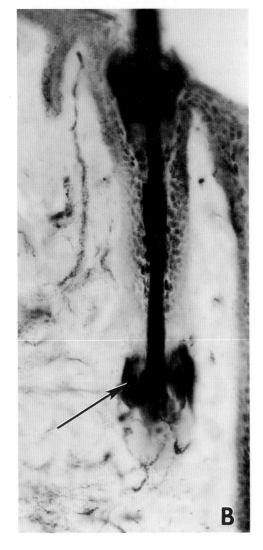

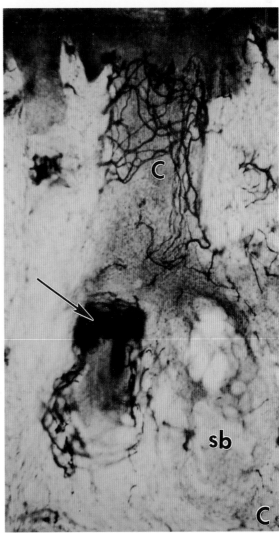

PLATE 106

NERVES
Hair Follicle

A. Numerous acetylcholinesterase-reactive nerves around the bulb of a hair (hr) follicle from the glabella (the space between the eyebrows and above the bridge of the nose). There are more nerves around the hair follicles in the eyebrows, glabella, eyelashes, and nose than in follicles anywhere else on the body. From a 20-year-old man. 40-μm frozen section. Koelle's acetylcholinesterase technique. OM 100x.

B. The follicles of the cilia (eyelashes) have myelinated nerve end organs (arrow) in which most of the nerve fibers are oriented horizontally, at right angles to the hair (hr) follicle. 30-μm frozen section. Winkelmann's nerve technique. OM 125x.

C. Nerve end organ (arrow) around a telogen vellus hair (hr) follicle in the periareolar area of the breast of a young woman. 20-μm frozen section. Winkelmann's nerve technique. OM 250x.

D. Nerve end organ (arrow) around a hair (hr) follicle in the glabella of a young man. Regardless of where hair follicle nerve end organs are found, they are similar. 20-μm frozen section. Winkelmann's nerve technique. OM 120x.

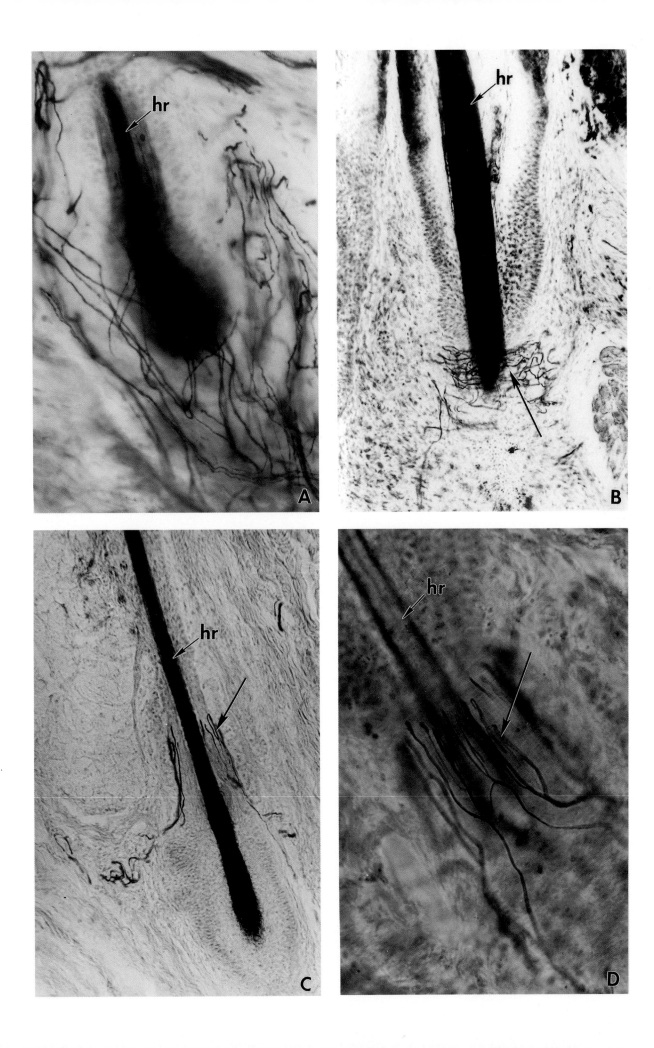

Glands

The glands, appendages of the skin, include:

1. Apocrine Glands
2. Eccrine Sweat Glands
3. Mixed Glands
4. Buccal Glands
5. Sebaceous Glands

Each type of gland has unique morphological characteristics and functions. All of these cutaneous appendages arise from the embryonic epidermis.

PLATE 107

APOCRINE GLANDS

Axillary Organ

This diagram shows a sebaceous gland, an apocrine gland, and an eccrine sweat gland around a hair follicle. These organs comprise the anatomical and functional units of the axillary organ. The axillary organ is a hominoid structure found only in the axilla of the chimpanzee, gorilla, and man.

Some of the largest skin glands are found in the axilla, a warm, moist skin fold that produces the distinctive human body odor. Secretions from the apocrine glands are dissolved by the watery eccrine sweat and spread over the axillary surface. Resident bacteria proliferate in this area and secrete enzymes that attack the apocrine secretion, releasing the typical odor.

The apocrine and eccrine glands, originally classified on the basis of their mode of secretion, are both known as "sweat" glands, but this is misleading. Apocrine glands were originally believed to secrete by a process in which the apical portion of the cytoplasm was sloughed off into the lumen. This type of secretion has been questioned. We now believe that all the mechanisms of exocrine glandular secretion, from merocrine to holocrine, may be at play in these glands. In addition, since human apocrine glands do not respond to thermal stimulation, their products should not be called "sweat."

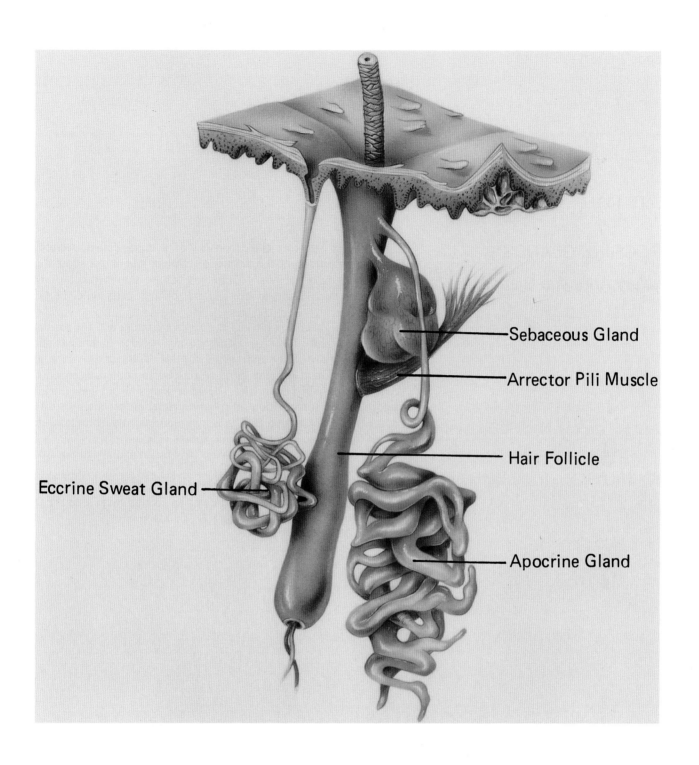

Sebaceous Gland

Arrector Pili Muscle

Hair Follicle

Apocrine Gland

Eccrine Sweat Gland

PLATE 108

APOCRINE GLANDS

Axillary Apocrine Glands

The tubular apocrine gland consists of a large, coiled, secretory portion embedded in the dermis or hypodermis and a short duct that opens into the pilary canal just above the entrance of the sebaceous duct. Some apocrine glands open directly onto the skin surface.

Apocrine glands are located mainly in the axilla and the perineal areas. The odor-producing glands do not become functional until puberty and are under androgenic control. The glands, which are small in children, become large and active in adolescence and remain functional in adult life. The odor wanes in old age. Little is known of the composition of apocrine secretion because it is difficult to collect secretion that is not contaminated with sebum and sweat from sebaceous and eccrine glands, respectively.

This SEM photograph shows a nearly intact axillary organ from a split-skin preparation of the axilla of a 20-year-old man. It contains a hair follicle (H), a sebaceous gland (S), an apocrine gland (A) and its duct (AD), and the duct of an eccrine sweat gland (ED). OM 100x. Courtesy of Dr. Dennis D. Knudson.

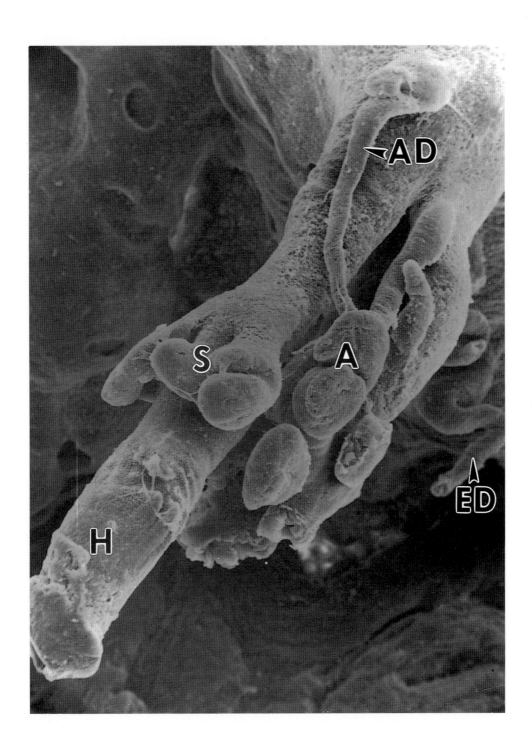

PLATE 109

APOCRINE GLANDS

Axillary Apocrine Glands

A. Apocrine gland secretory tubules from the axilla of a middle-aged Black man are lined with columnar epithelium with large spherical nuclei near the bases of the cells. The shape and size of the secretory cells in the tubules are variable and reflect the cells' activity. Lumen (L). 2-μm plastic section. H and Lee. OM 160x.

B. This tubule from the same section as in Figure A is lined with cuboidal secretory cells with large nuclei. The cytoplasm of the cells is packed with secretory granules (G). The tubule is surrounded by a thin basement membrane and a thick connective tissue capsule. Lumen (L). H and Lee. OM 630x.

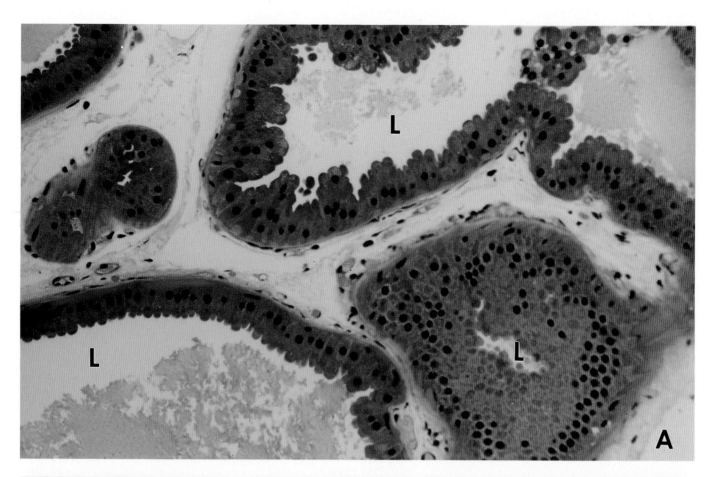

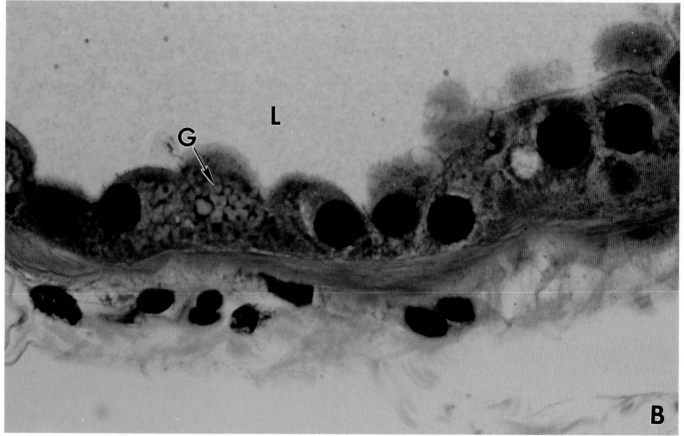

PLATE 110

APOCRINE GLANDS

Axillary Apocrine Glands

A. Axillary apocrine gland stained with a mixture of sirius red and sirius blue, pH 2.0, which stains proteinaceous substances. The secretory cells have a basal nucleus, above which is a prominent negative image of the Golgi complex (G). Lumen (L). 2-μm plastic section. OM 160x.

B. The cells of the apocrine glands in the axillary skin of a 36-year-old man are replete with secretory granules (S) around the nucleus. The cells have a convex luminal border. The apical cytoplasm contains no discrete granules. Above the nuclei, with their prominent nucleoli, are the negative images of the Golgi bodies (G). The epithelial cells rest upon a myoepithelial cell (M). Collagenous capsule (C). Lumen (L). 2-μm plastic section. Sirius red and sirius blue, pH 2.0. OM 1200x.

C. Tubule of an apocrine gland from the axilla of a 20-year-old man, stained with a technique that shows elastic fibers (E). The secretory epithelium contains pigmented granules that stain a reddish color. The overall yellow color is nonspecific staining from the orange G in the staining mixture. The sloughed cells in the lumen (L) also contain reddish-colored secretory granules. 20-μm frozen section. Roman's AOV elastic fiber technique. OM 250x.

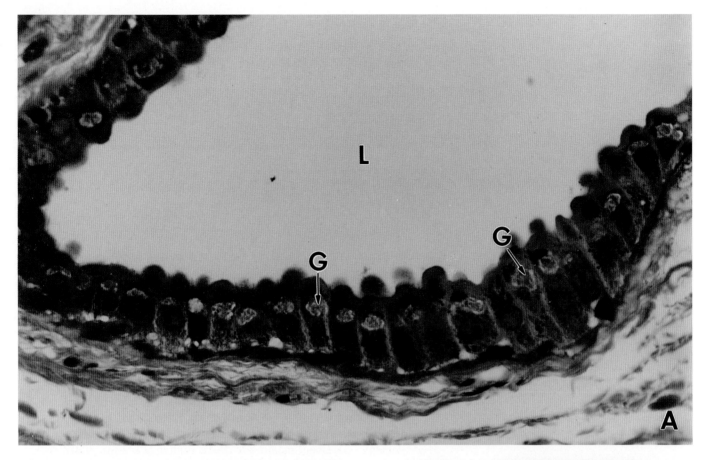

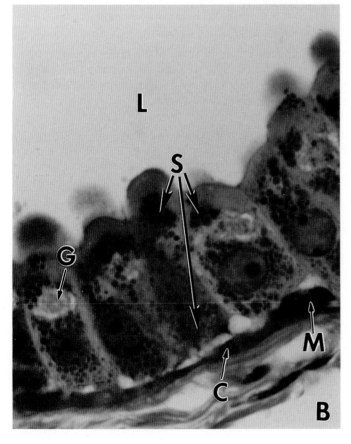

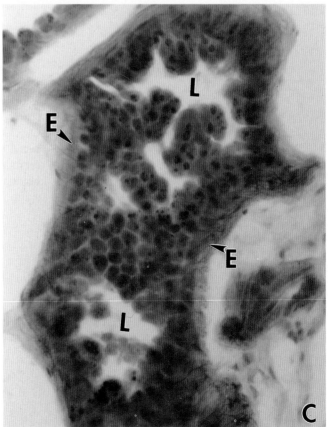

PLATE 111

APOCRINE GLANDS

Axillary Apocrine Glands

The secretory cells from the axilla of a 36-year-old man have been stained with Giemsa. The variability in the appearance of the secretory epithelium may be indicative of a great range in secretory activity of the cells.

A. Low columnar cells line one of the tubules. Small secretory granules (SG) are scattered throughout the cells. The clear area above the nucleus is the negative image of the Golgi area (G). The secretory epithelium is surrounded by myoepithelial cells (M) that are cut both transversely and longitudinally. The myoepithelial cells may be contractile and responsible for fluctuations in the rate of production of the apocrine glands, or they may be sustentacular elements. Basement membrane (BM). Lumen (L). 2-μm plastic section. Giemsa stain. OM 630x.

B. Columnar cells with conspicuous secretory blebs (SB) are characteristic of active apocrine glands. Some of the blebs appear to be detached. Secretory granules (SG) are clustered around the Golgi area (G). Myoepithelial cells (M) are cut longitudinally. Lumen (L). 2-μm plastic section. Giemsa stain. OM 630x.

C. Cells are cast off (CO) into the lumen (L) and contribute to the secretory product. Thus, axillary apocrine glands show holocrine secretion as well as eccrine and apocrine types of secretion. Myoepithelial cells (M). Blood vessel (BV). 2-μm plastic section. Giemsa stain. OM 630x.

D. Some secretory tubules or even entire glands may be swollen and lined with very flat secretory cells. The lumen (L) contains a flocculent material (FM), which may have visible cell debris. Myoepithelial cell (M). 2-μm plastic section. Giemsa stain. OM 630x.

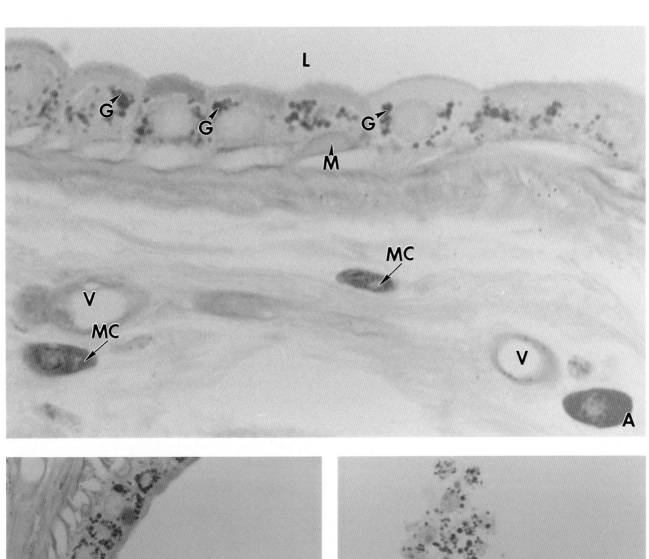

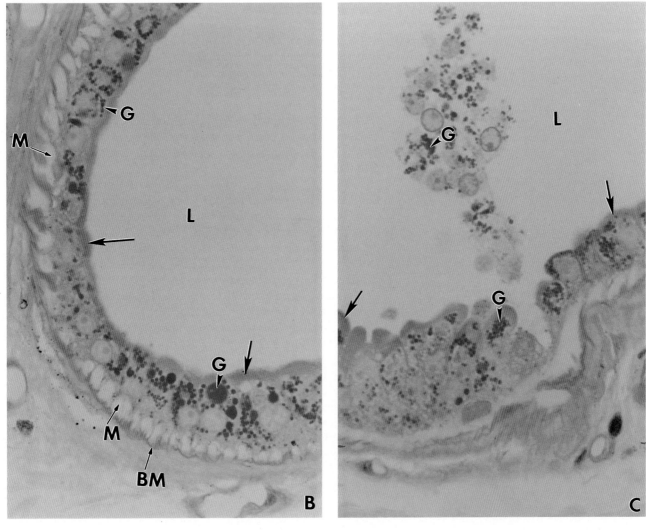

PLATE 114

APOCRINE GLANDS

Axillary Apocrine Glands

A. Masses of apocrine glands (AG) in the axillary skin of a 20-year-old man are much larger than the clusters of eccrine sweat gland (EG) tubules. Apocrine glands respond to adrenomimetic stimuli only after puberty and can be stimulated by either epinephrine or norepinephrine. Hair follicles (HF) have been cut transversely in this section. H & E 30-μm frozen section. OM 25x. Courtesy of Dr. Hideo Uno. From D. Robertshaw, "Apocrine Sweat Glands," in *Biochemistry and Physiology of Skin, Vol. I*, editor L. Goldsmith, by permission of Oxford University Press, 1983. New York.

B. Sparse acetylcholinesterase-reactive nerves around the axillary apocrine glands (AG) contrast with the tightly wound nerves around the eccrine sweat glands (EG), which are controlled primarily by cholinergic nerves. 20-μm frozen section. Koelle's acetylcholinesterase technique. OM 63x. Courtesy of Dr. Hideo Uno. From D. Robertshaw, "Apocrine Sweat Glands," in *Biochemistry and Physiology of Skin, Vol. I*, editor L. Goldsmith, by permission of Oxford University Press, 1983. New York.

C. In contrast with those in the axilla, thick acetylcholinesterase-reactive nerves are conspicuous around the apocrine glands of Moll in the eyelids. 20-μm frozen section. Koelle's acetylcholinesterase technique. OM 120x.

D. TEM micrograph of the cells of an axillary apocrine gland with many large secretory granules (G) around the nucleus (N). There are no granules in the apical cytoplasm. Myoepithelial cells (M) are at the base of the secretory cells. Courtesy of Dr. Hideo Uno.

E. Nerve fibers (N) around a secretory tubule of an apocrine gland. The terminal axon profiles (arrows) in the periglandular collagenous tissue contain mostly agranular vesicles. An intact nerve supply is a functional requirement for apocrine secretion. Myoepithelial cell (M). Lumen (L). OM 3500x. Courtesy of Dr. Hideo Uno.

F. Nerve terminal around a tubule of an axillary apocrine gland. The nerve contains small, agranular vesicles (arrowheads) and large, dense-cored vesicles (arrows) typical of cholinergic nerves. Unmyelinated fibers have been found close to capillaries; the capillary circulation assists in transporting transmitter substances to the apocrine gland cells. OM 44,000x. Courtesy of Dr. Hideo Uno.

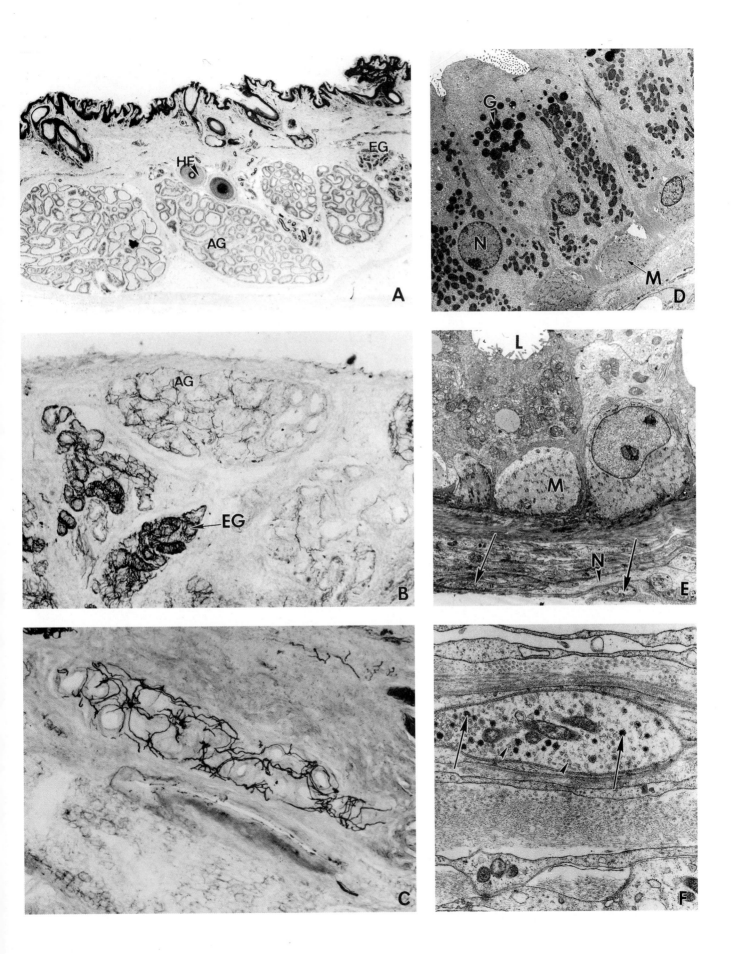

PLATE 115

APOCRINE GLANDS

Axillary Apocrine Glands

A. Low-power SEM micrograph of a cut tubule of an axillary apocrine gland. The loose connective tissue (Ct) between the tubules holds them in place. Each gland is embedded in a tight connective tissue sheath. OM 350x. Reprinted by permission of VCH Publishers, Inc., 220 East 23rd St., New York, N.Y. 10010 from Wilborn, Hyde and Montes, *SEM of Normal and Abnormal Human Skin*, p. 112. 1985.

B. SEM micrograph of an axillary apocrine tubule. The surface of the secretory cells is covered with microvilli. Clear blebs (B), the secretory protrusions,extend from some cells into the lumen. OM 2290x. Reprinted by permission of VCH Publishers, Inc., 220 East 23rd St., New York, N.Y. 10010 from Wilborn, Hyde and Montes, *SEM of Normal and Abnormal Human Skin*, p. 112. 1985.

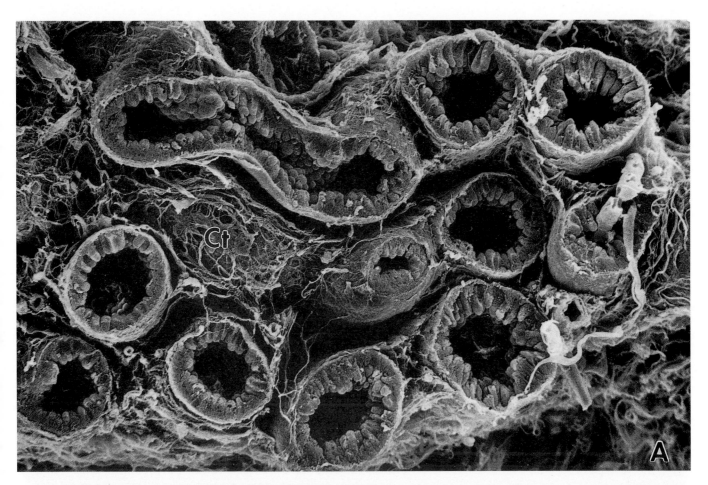

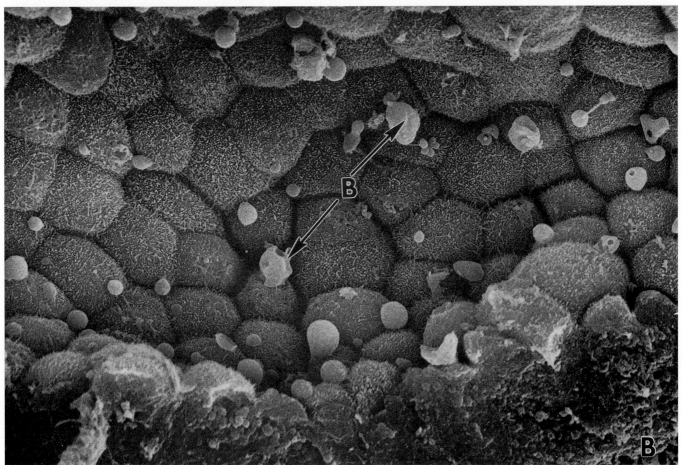

PLATE 116

APOCRINE GLANDS

Axillary Apocrine Glands

A. Holocrine secretion results in cell loss; the remaining cells may divide to repopulate the tubules. This is an axillary apocrine gland cell dividing (metaphase). Note the spindle fibers (arrow) that are attached to the chromosomes (C). 5-μm paraffin section. Regaud's iron hematoxylin. OM 1200x.

B. Distinct, blue-stained, ionic iron-containing lipofuschin pigment granules (arrow) in a columnar secretory epithelium in an axillary apocrine gland. The active glands of some individuals, however, can be free of pigment and/or iron. Lumen (L). 4-μm plastic section. Pearl's Prussian blue iron technique. OM 630x.

C. Many cells of this tubule have iron-containing pigment granules (arrow); adjacent cells are free of them. Intraepithelial ionic iron is a distinctive feature of some apocrine glands. From the axilla of a 20-year-old White man. 10-μm paraffin section. Pearl's Prussian blue iron technique. OM 630x.

D. Apocrine secretory cells contain only dust-like particles reactive to Hale's colloidal iron technique. A dense blue band at the periphery (arrows) and the material inside the lumen (L) are stained. From the axilla of a 36-year-old man. 2-μm plastic section. Hale's colloidal iron technique. OM 400x.

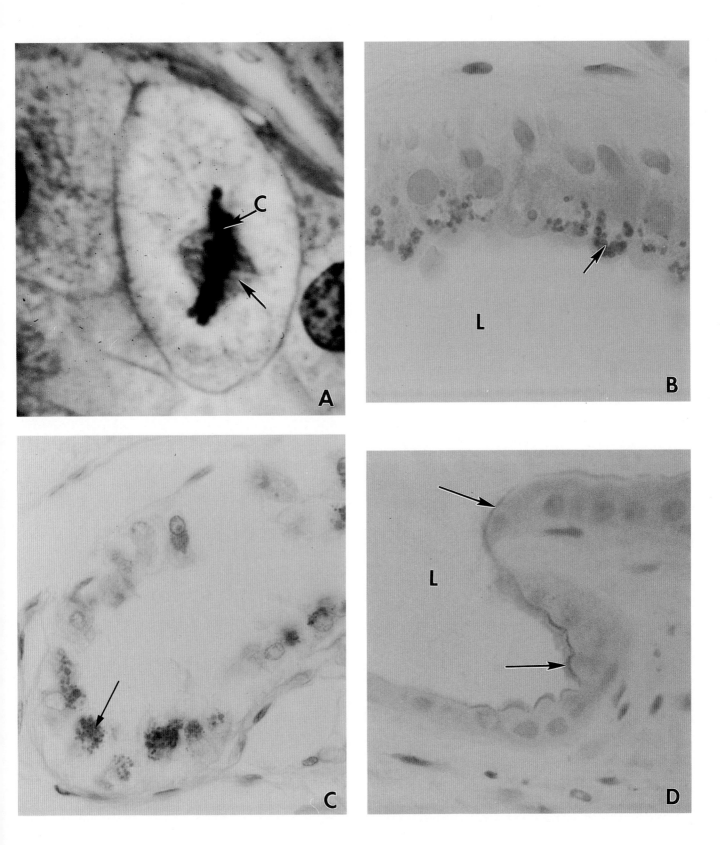

PLATE 117

APOCRINE GLANDS
Axillary Apocrine Glands

A. Tubule from the axillary gland of a young White man. Fine elastic fibers (arrows) surround the tubules. Secretory granules (G). Lumen (L). 4-μm plastic section. Verhoff's elastic fiber technique. OM 250x.

B. Axillary apocrine gland surrounded by a very fine web of elastic fibers (arrows). 20-μm frozen section. Roman's AOV elastic fiber technique. OM 630x.

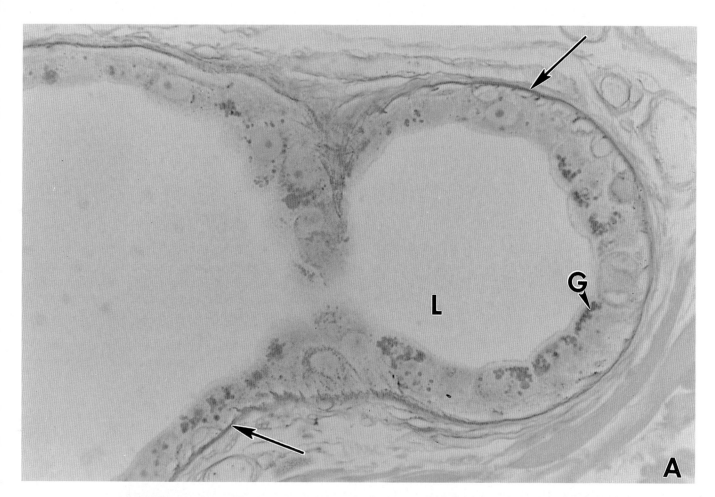

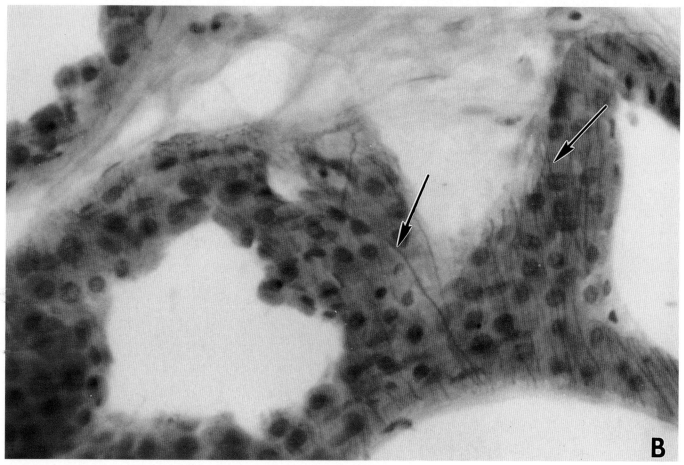

PLATE 118

APOCRINE GLANDS

Axillary Apocrine Glands

A. The axilla of a middle-aged Black man shows apocrine glands (A), mixed glands (M), eccrine sweat glands (E), and a mucous gland (Mc). Mucous glands are frequently encountered in the axilla of Black people. 2-μm plastic section. H and Lee. OM 160x.

B. Enlargement of the mucous gland shown in Figure A. The gland is surrounded by a basement membrane (arrow), outside of which is a thick collagenous fiber capsule (C). 2-μm plastic section. H and Lee. OM 250x.

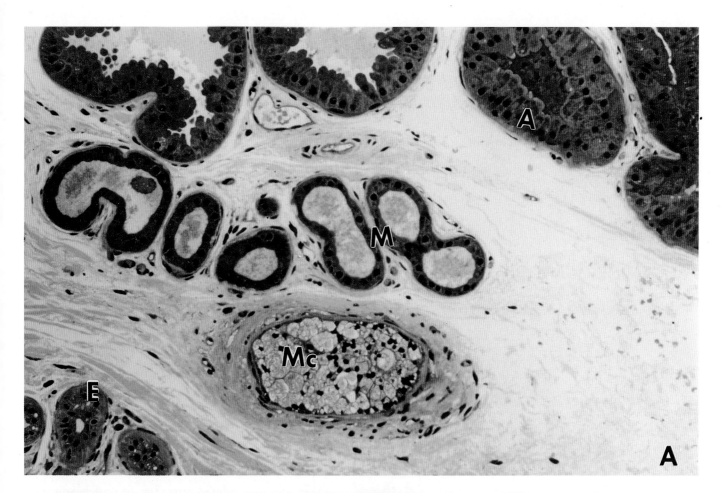

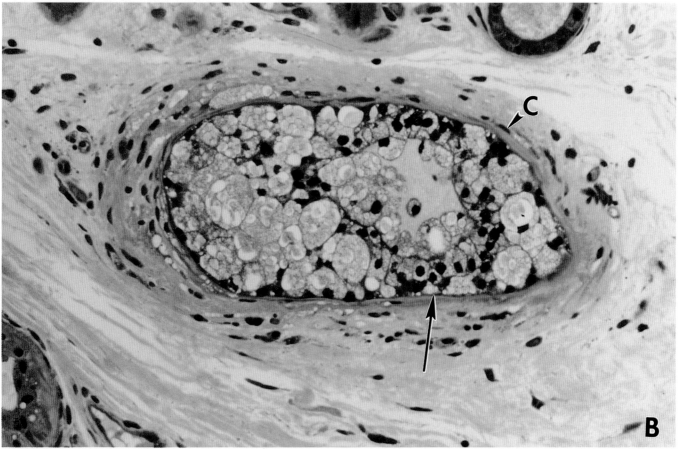

PLATE 119

APOCRINE GLANDS

Facial Apocrine Glands

A. The upper part of the apocrine secretory segment (A) narrows and emerges into a duct (D) that opens into the pilary canal (PC) of a nearby hair follicle above the entrance of a sebaceous gland (S) in the face of a middle-aged White woman. Although such glands have been dubbed "ectopic" (meaning aberrant or out of place), they often occur in the facial skin and scalp of people of all races, a reflection of their fetal development in association with a hair follicle. 2-μm plastic section. H and Lee. OM 160x.

B. Cross section of the duct (D) of an apocrine gland embedded in the upper part of a hair follicle (HF) in the face of a young White woman. Sebaceous gland (S). 2-μm plastic section. H and Lee. OM 250x.

C. Typical apocrine secretory tubules from the face of a young White woman. 2-μm plastic section. H and Lee. OM 250x.

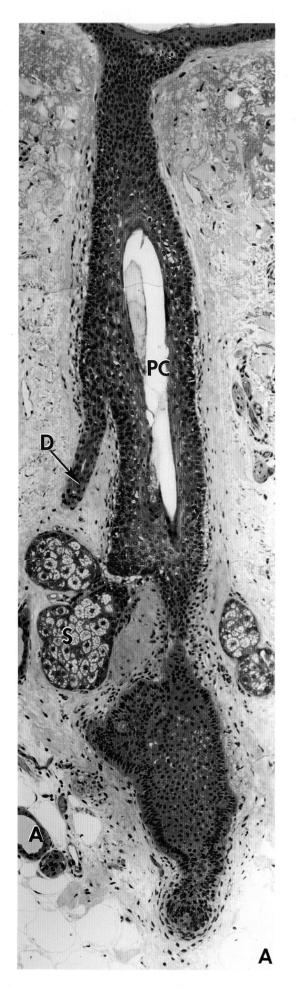

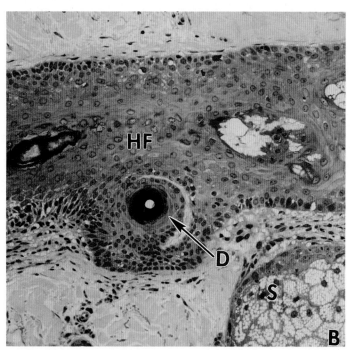

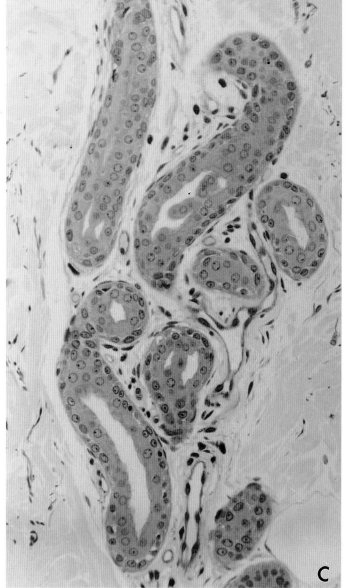

PLATE 120

ECCRINE SWEAT GLANDS
Surface

Sweating, the normal response to exercise, heat, and emotional stress, is the secretion of water and electrolytes onto the surface of the skin. Sweat is intimately associated with the blood vascular system as the principal modulator of body temperature. Sweating also keeps the skin damp; a dry hand or foot has poor grip and sensibility.

More than three million eccrine sweat glands are distributed over the body, but there is great individual variation in gland density. In adult bodies, the palms and soles have the most sweat glands. Sweat glands develop in the palms and soles of the fetus during the third month and in the axilla during the fifth month; later they appear over the rest of the body.

A. This photograph shows a loop pattern of dermatoglyphics in the index finger of a young person. At the apex of each ridge are the pores of sweat glands (arrows). In the hands of young people one can often see sweat inside the pores, and as Marcello Malpighi (1628–1694) noted, the level of the liquid is constantly rising or falling. OM 16x. Courtesy of Prof. Antonio Tosti.

B. Bubbles of sweat emerge from the pores at the summit of the ridges on the thumb of a young man. Sweating controls body temperature through evaporative heat loss. There is great variation in the amount of sweating that is stimulated by stress. Some persons sweat profusely, while others sweat little. Individual differences in sweating cannot always be explained by such factors as sex or age. When this mechanism fails, hyperthermia and death can result. OM 16x. Courtesy of Prof. Antonio Tosti.

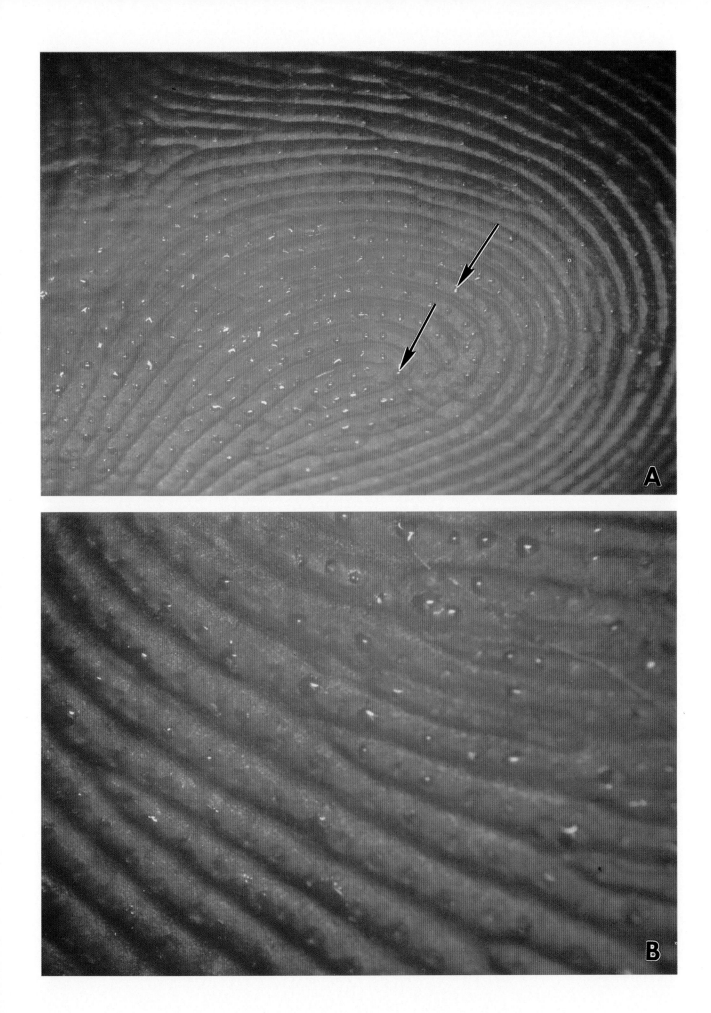

PLATE 121

ECCRINE SWEAT GLANDS

Surface

A. SEM micrograph of dermatoglyphic ridges with sweat bubbles in the pores. The openings of the sweat ducts (arrows) look like suction cups when they do not cradle a sweat bubble. The "pores" may indeed function as suction cups. OM 50x. Courtesy of Dr. W. H. Fahrenbach.

B. SEM micrograph of the opening of a sweat gland in the palm of a young Black woman. The opening has a helical shape and resembles the inside of a snail shell. Sweating on the palms and soles is fairly continuous when a person is awake. The sweating triggered by emotional stress is most profuse on the palms, soles, axilla, and forehead but can also occur over the entire body. OM 1000x. Courtesy of Dr. W. H. Fahrenbach.

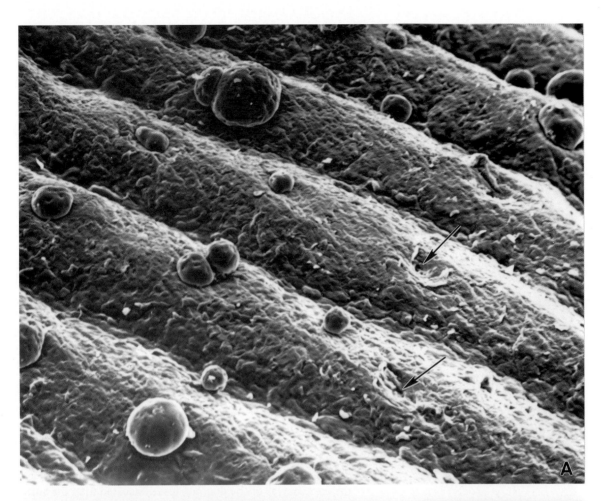

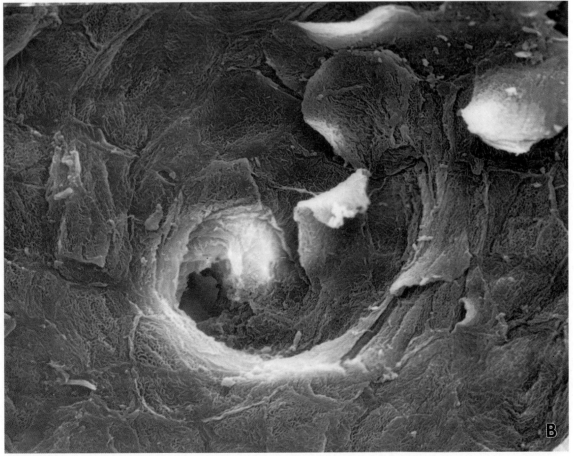

PLATE 122

ECCRINE SWEAT GLANDS

Sweat Duct

The eccrine duct consists of (1) a coiled proximal segment that is continuous with the secretory tubule, (2) a relatively straight distal segment, and (3) the acrosyringium or intraepidermal sweat duct unit. The main function of the duct is reabsorption of sodium from the secretory product with the production of hypotonic sweat. The reabsorption of water, salts, and electrolytes is vital for the maintenance of the body's homeostasis during excessive perspiration.

A. Duct of an eccrine sweat gland as it winds through the thin epidermis of the trunk of a young man. Both the duct cells and the adjacent keratinocytes retain their individuality in the epidermal sweat-duct unit. The duct cells usually contain little or no pigment, in contrast with those of the surrounding epidermis. The coiled duct is cut several times (arrowheads) in the stratum corneum where the corneocytes of the duct are less desiccated than the surrounding stratum corneum cells. 2-μm plastic section. H and Lee. OM 160x.

B. The terminal portion of a sweat duct winds through the palmar epidermis of an 18-year-old woman. 2-μm plastic section. H and Lee. OM 250x.

C. Transverse section of the duct of an eccrine sweat gland just before it enters the epidermis of the trunk of a young woman. The duct has two to four layers of cells. The basal cells contain glycogen granules (G). The cornified luminal cells (C) form the cuticular border. Basement membrane (BM). 4-μm plastic section. PAS. OM 1000x.

D. Transverse sections of the coiled proximal segments of a sweat gland duct in the hand of a young woman. More active reabsorption occurs in this portion of the duct than in the distal segment. Glycogen granules (G) are numerous in the basal cells. Cuticular border (C). The section of the duct on the right is closer to the secretory tubule than the one on the left; the cuticular border is not well formed in this duct segment. Note the prominent PAS-reactive basement membrane (BM). Epithelial cells everywhere sit upon a basement membrane that is thought to regulate transfer of nutrients. 4-μm plastic section. PAS. OM 1000x.

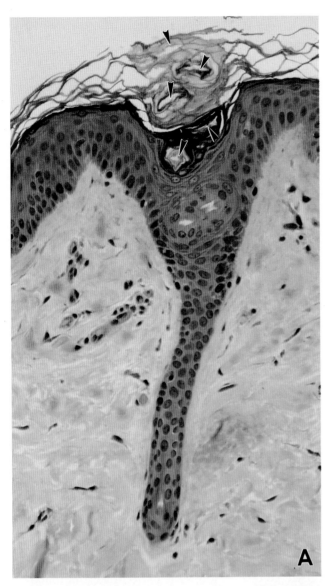
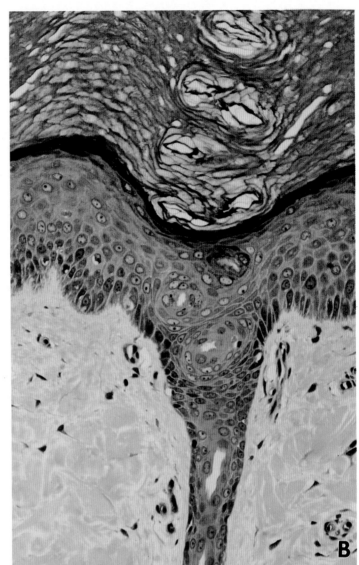
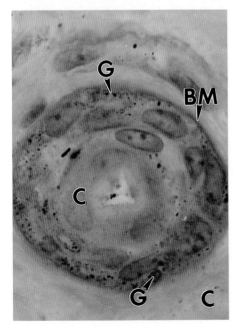
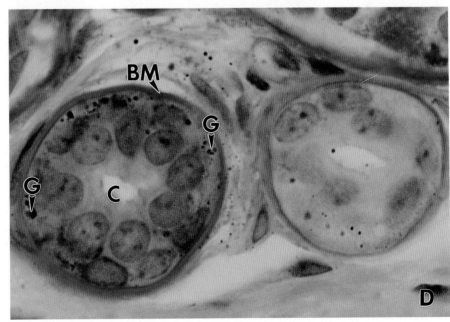

PLATE 123

ECCRINE SWEAT GLANDS

Eccrine Secretory Tubule

The secretory epithelium of the sweat glands is usually composed of three distinct cell types: (1) clear cells, (2) dark cells, and (3) myoepithelial cells. The dark cells border nearly all the luminal surface of the tubules. There are, however, some glands whose secretory cells differ from both clear and dark cells.

A. Transverse section of a secretory segment and a duct (Dt) from the arm of a young man. In this secretory epithelium, the dark cells (D) are full of secretory granules that stain with basic dyes. These cells are cuboidal and appear to rest on top of the clear cells, or they appear as inverted pyramidal cells whose cytoplasmic processes extend downward between clear cells. The cytoplasm of clear cells (C) stains faintly with basic dyes. Myoepithelial cells (M) form the outermost layer of the secretory tubule. The function of myoepithelial cells is not known; they may contract or act as a structural support for the gland. 2-μm plastic section. Toluidine blue, pH 5.0. OM 630x.

B. Sections of an eccrine sweat gland from the trunk of a young Black woman. Sweat gland secretory cells are delicate and are easily distorted when fixed. In this section, secretory cells contain round vacuoles in their cytoplasm and have a reticulated appearance. They are neither clear nor dark cells. In some people, all of the eccrine glands are lined with vacuolated and reticulated secretory cells. 2-μm plastic section. Giemsa stain. OM 630x.

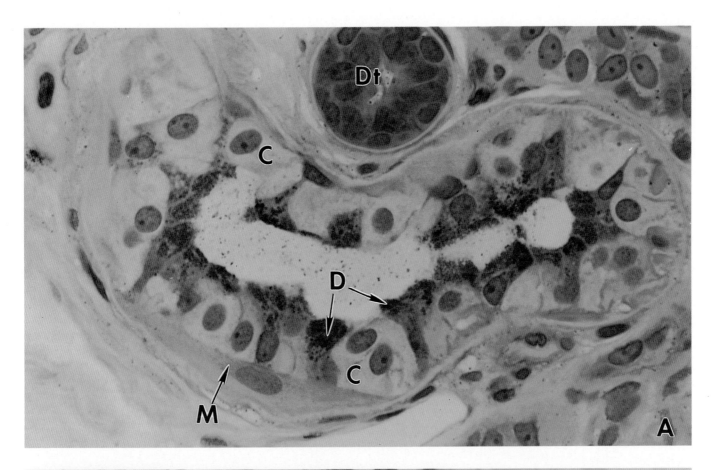

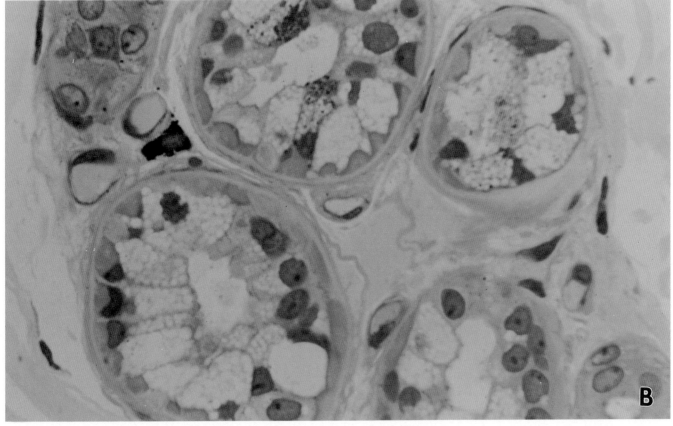

PLATE 124

ECCRINE SWEAT GLANDS

Eccrine Secretory Tubule

A. Transverse sections through an eccrine sweat gland showing clear cells (C) laden with glycogen granules, and dark cells (D) with few or no visible granules. With this technique, "clear" cells appear red and "dark" cells appear clear. Basement membrane (BM). 4-μm plastic section. PAS. OM 630x.

B. Sparse PAS-reactive material (arrows) in reticulated secretory cells of eccrine sweat glands from the trunk skin of a young Black woman. Some normal clear cells (C) are replete with glycogen granules. Basement membrane (BM). 2-μm plastic section. PAS. OM 250x.

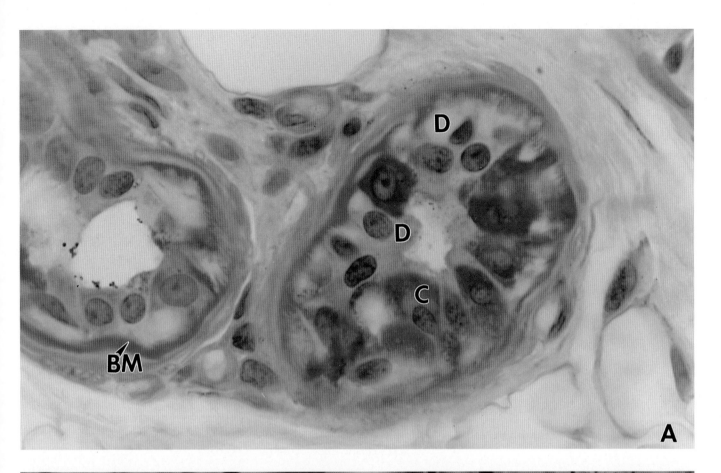

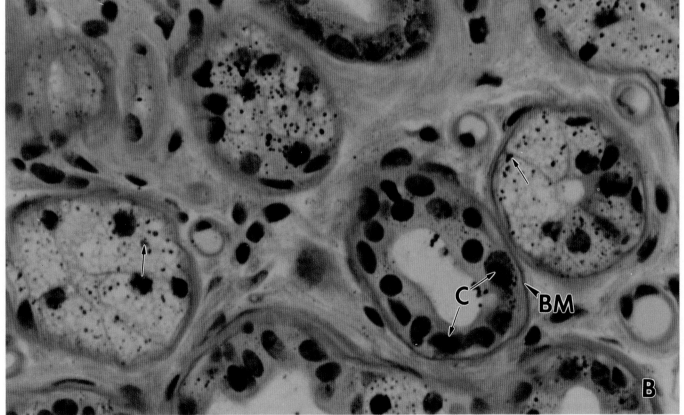

PLATE 125

ECCRINE SWEAT GLANDS

Elastic Fibers

Aging

A. This eccrine sweat gland has been teased from the axillary skin of a young woman; the thinner, darker-stained coiled duct (arrow) reacts strongly for succinic dehydrogenase, an oxidative mitochondrial enzyme. The ductal cells, which reabsorb sodium, are known to be rich in mitochondria. Succinic dehydrogenase technique. OM 50x.

B. Elastic fibers are tightly wrapped around the secretory portion of an eccrine sweat gland from the axilla of a young man. Few elastic fibers surround the coiled segment of the duct. 30-μm frozen section. Roman's AOV elastic fiber technique. OM 650x.

C. Layer of fine elastic fibers (E) around an eccrine sweat gland from the face of a middle-aged woman. 4-μm plastic section. Weigert's elastic fiber technique. OM 630x.

D. Elastic fibers (E) seem to have increased in amount and in coarseness around the secretory coil of a sweat gland in the photo-damaged face of a 70-year-old man. Excessive deposition of elastin, commonly called "elastosis," is characteristic of old, actinically damaged skin. 4-μm plastic section. Weigert's elastic fiber technique. OM 630x.

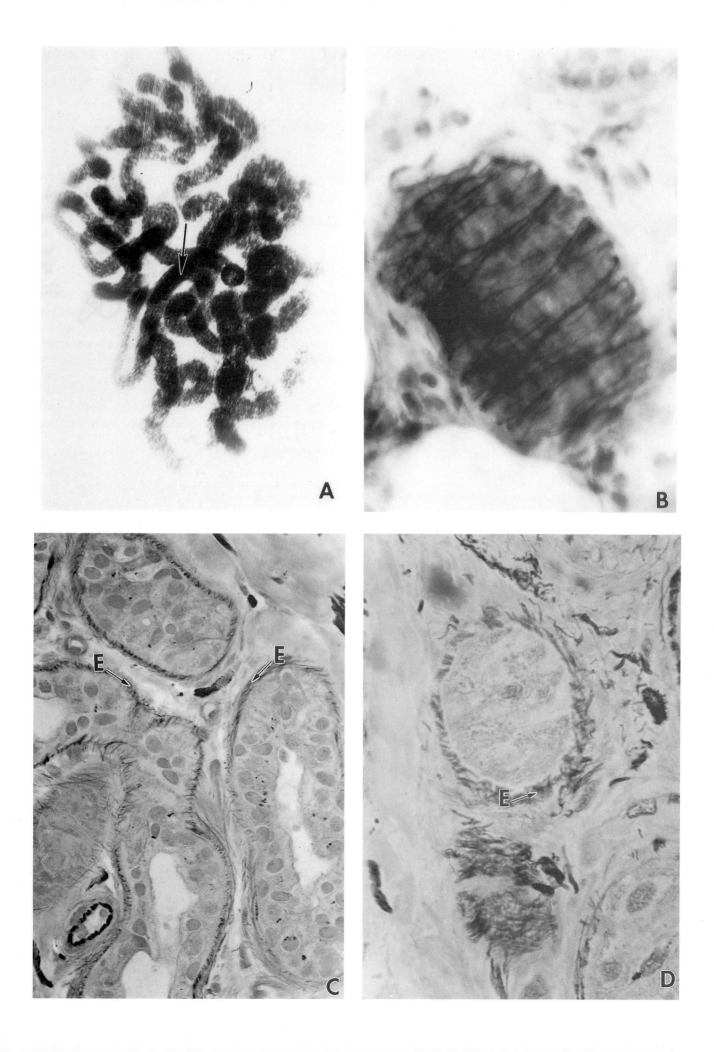

PLATE 126

ECCRINE SWEAT GLANDS
Nerves

Regulation of body temperature is the most important function of sweat. Efferent nerve fibers from the preoptic sweat center of the hypothalamus descend through the brain stem and spinal tract. The nerves that surround the eccrine sweat glands are nonmyelinated fibers of the sympathetic postganglionic nerves.

A. The entire tubule of the eccrine sweat gland is surrounded by fine cholinesterase-reactive nerves. There are many more nerves around the secretory coil (S) than around the nearby coiled duct (D). From the axilla of a 20-year-old man. Koelle's acetylcholinesterase technique. OM 100x.

B. Tightly wound cholinesterase-reactive nerves around the secretory coils of eccrine glands. From the axilla of a young woman. 20-μm frozen section. Koelle's acetylcholinesterase technique. OM 100x.

C. Both cholinergic and adrenergic nerves have been demonstrated around eccrine sweat glands. Fluorescent catecholamine-containing nerves around the secretory tubules of an eccrine sweat gland from the axilla of a young man are demonstrated with a histofluorescent technique that shows the presence of catecholamines. Eccrine sweat glands respond primarily to cholinergic drugs, but they also respond to adrenergic drugs. OM 250x. Courtesy of Dr. H. Uno.

D. Nonmyelinated nerves (N) near the basal lamina (BL) of an eccrine sweat gland. There are dense granules and vesicles inside the nerves. Note the interdigitations between clear cells (C), and a large intercellular canaliculus (IC). OM 12,000x. Courtesy of Prof. Ken Hashimoto.

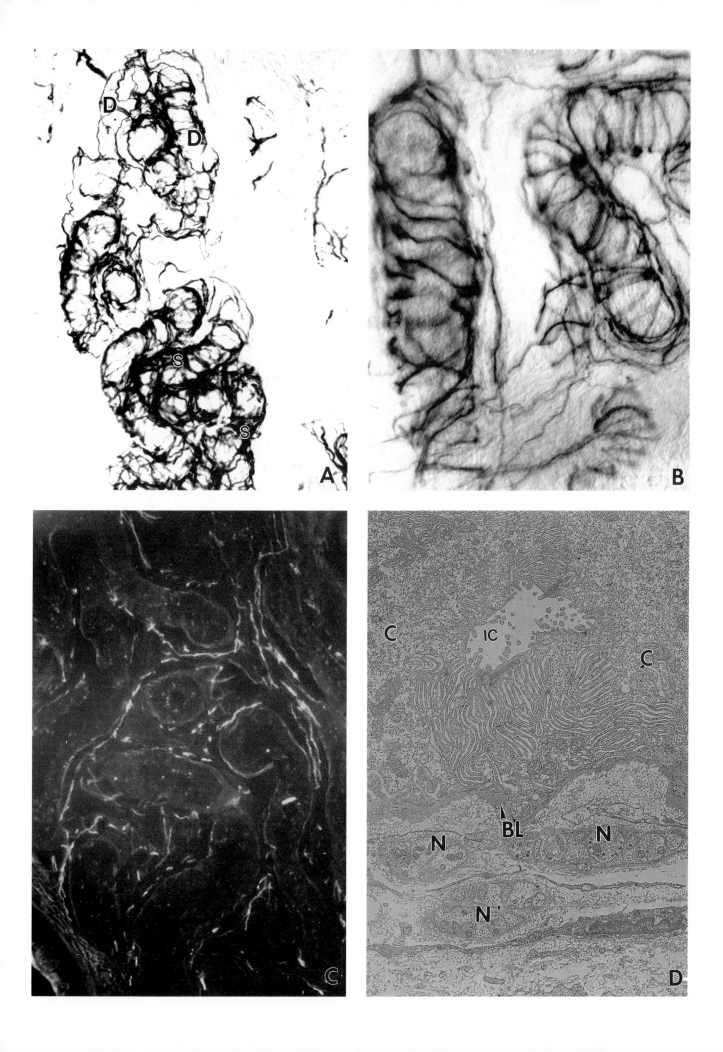

PLATE 127

ECCRINE SWEAT GLANDS

A. TEM of a transverse section through an eccrine gland. Clear cells (C) are responsible for secretion of water and electrolytes. They contain numerous mitochondria and secretory granules. The slender dark cells (D), which secrete what has been called a mucoid substance, extend from the myoepithelial cells (M) to the glandular lumen. OM 7750x. Courtesy of Dr. Mary Bell.

B. TEM of a transverse section of a secretory tubule. Dark cells (D) contain immature granules (I) and smaller, dark, mature granules (M). The granules vary in appearance according to their state of maturity. The luminal border of the dark-cell plasma membrane forms short microvilli. Clear cells (C) form an intricate system of intercellular canaliculi (arrows) with adjacent clear cells. Myoepithelial (Me) cell. OM 4,320x. Reprinted by permission of VCH Publishers, Inc., 220 East 23rd St., New York, N.Y. 10010 from Wilborn, Hyde and Montes, *SEM of Normal and Abnormal Human Skin*, p. 110. 1985.

C. TEM of interdigitating (I) plasma membranes of adjacent clear cells. Intercellular canaliculi (IC) are formed where two or more clear cells come in contact. The canaliculi open directly into the glandular lumen. Courtesy of Dr. Mary Bell.

D. The channels between clear cells can be demonstrated by deposits of lanthanum, which outlines the tortuous course of intercellular spaces. The channels open into the lumen (L) of the secretory coil. The luminal end of the intercellular space is broken up by tight junctions. The clear cell (C) on the right of the lanthanum-filled canaliculus contains rosettes of glycogen particles (G), mitochondria (M), and vesicles. The dark cell (D) contains a few glycogen particles and many dense granules (Gr), some fused with the luminal plasma membrane (arrowheads). OM 48,750x. Courtesy of Prof. Ken Hashimoto.

E. TEM of an intercellular canaliculus (IC) nearly filled with the villi of surrounding secretory cells that rest on myoepithelial cells (M). The clear cells contain small vesicles (V) along the luminal plasma membrane. The lanthanum-filled intercellular spaces are deeply infolded, forming interdigitations that hold the cells firmly together. Similarly, the basal parts of the clear cells form complex, long folds that interdigitate with those of adjacent clear cells. Microtubules (arrow). OM 21,000x. Courtesy of Prof. Ken Hashimoto.

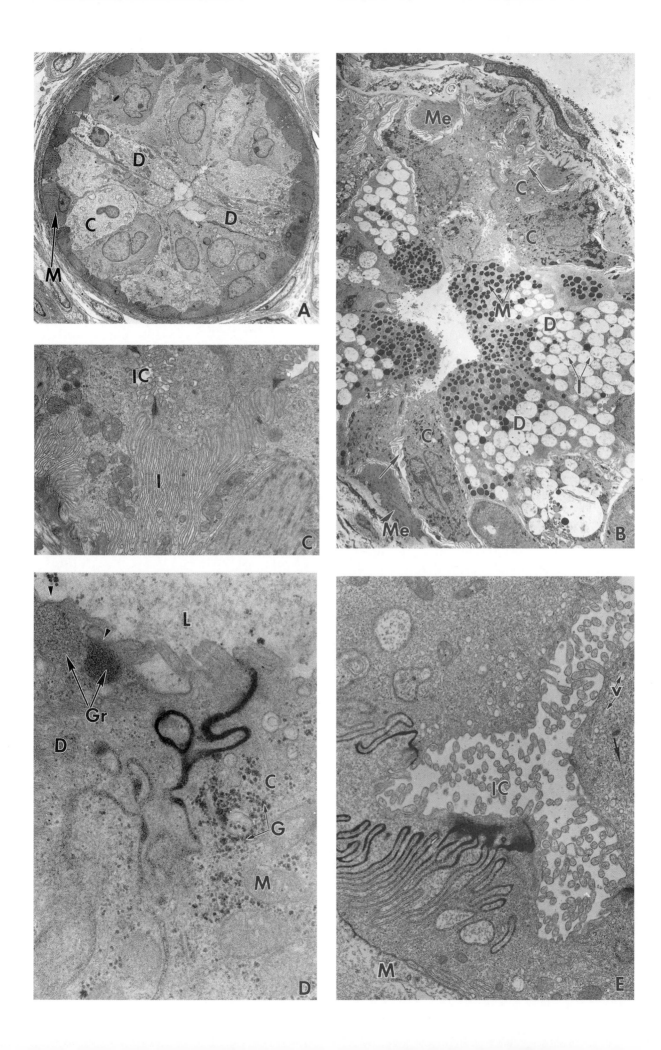

PLATE 128

ECCRINE SWEAT GLANDS
Aging Changes

In both exposed and unexposed skin, the eccrine secretory tubule shows aging changes. These changes may partially account for the decreased sweating in elderly men.

A. In aged persons, the secretory tubule of the sweat glands can undergo variable degeneration and shrinkage. In this section of the trunk skin of a 75-year-old White man, the tubules have disappeared, leaving only segments of coiled duct. This duct shows increased cornification of the luminal cells (L) and vacuolated basal cells (B). The blood vessels (BV) are dilated and full of red blood corpuscles. 2-µm plastic section. H and Lee. OM 1000x.

B. These transverse sections of an eccrine sweat gland from the trunk of a 73-year-old man show a number of aging changes. The secretory cells have more pigment (P) than do those in younger skin; the cells are reticulated and vacuolated; and there is a great deal of atypia. The intercellular canaliculi (C) are ballooned. Basement membrane (BM). Duct (D). Dilated blood vessel (BV). 2-µm plastic section. H and Lee. OM 1000x.

C. Sweat gland in the severely sun-damaged face of a 70-year-old man. Pigment (P) is abundant and most of the secretory cells are vacuolated. Dilated intercellular canaliculi (C). Basement membrane (BM). Dilated blood vessels (BV). 2-µm plastic section. H and Lee. OM 1000x.

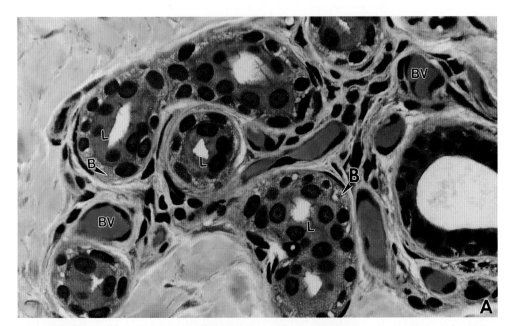

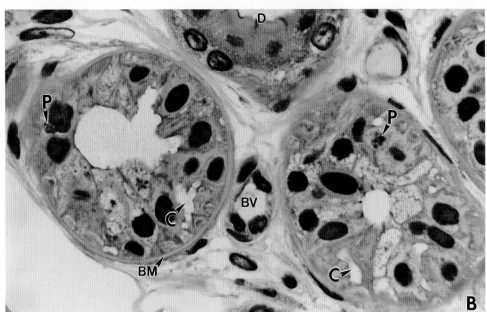

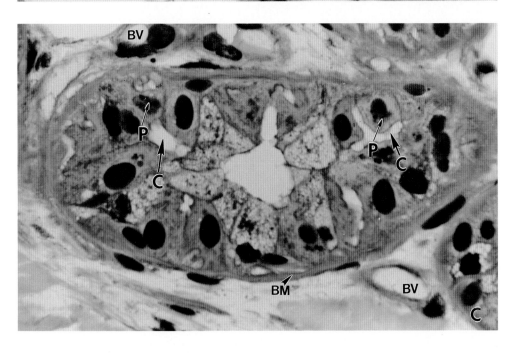

PLATE 129

MIXED GLANDS
Black Skin

Some glands, including those in the axilla, appear to be mixtures of apocrine and eccrine glands that open directly onto the surface of the skin. Mixed glands are more numerous in Black than in White skin. There is some controversy about the existence of mixed glands because of fixation artifacts, but close scrutiny of sweat glands in various histological preparations shows that (a) the structure of sweat glands needs to be reevaluated and (b) mixed apocrine–eccrine glands do exist.

A. This portion of a mixed apocrine–eccrine gland, from the skin of the face of a young Black woman, has apocrine-like cells (A) full of granules and reticulated cells (R) similar to those found in some eccrine glands. Myoepithelial cell (M). 2-μm plastic section. H and Lee. OM 750x.

B. Binucleated cells are common in mixed apocrine–eccrine glands in the face of a 42-year-old Black woman. These tubules are lined primarily with apocrine-like cells. Myoepithelial cell (M). 2-μm plastic section. H and Lee. OM 750x.

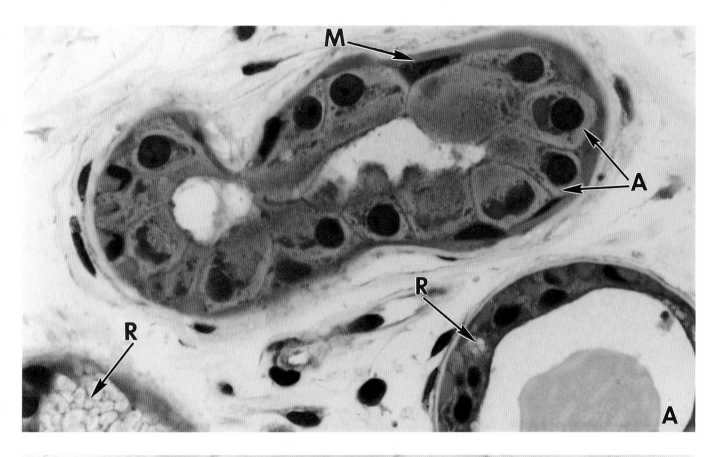

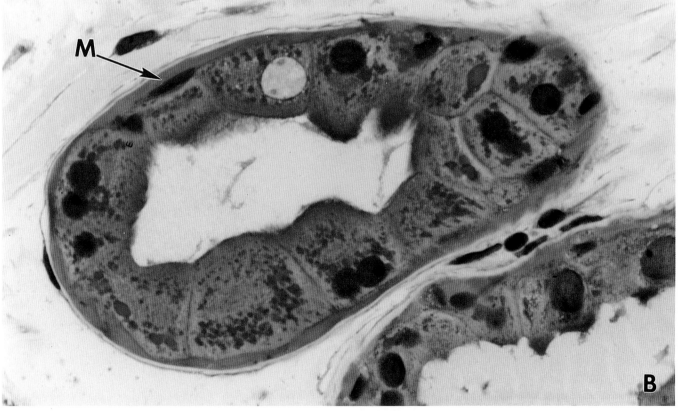

PLATE 130

MIXED GLANDS

PAS

A. These tubules of mixed glands from the facial skin of a young Black woman are lined with apocrine-like cells (A) as well as with vacuolated and reticulated eccrine-like cells (R). The lumen of the tubule on the right contains a dense mass of strongly PAS-reactive material. In the lumen of the tubule on the left, PAS-reactive material is sparse and granular. The pigment granules (arrowheads) are also PAS-reactive, as is the pigment in eccrine sweat glands, but they are inside apocrine-like cells. Basement membrane (BM). Myoepithelial cells (M). 4-μm plastic section. PAS. OM 630x.

B. This segment of a mixed gland is lined with apocrine-like cells and vacuolated, reticulated, eccrine-like cells (R). The apocrine cells have a PAS-reactive brush border (arrowhead). The tubules are surrounded by a PAS-reactive basement membrane (BM) outside of which is a collagenous capsule. The secretory cells rest on a layer of myoepithelial cells (M). PAS counterstained with hematoxylin. 4-μm plastic section. OM 630x.

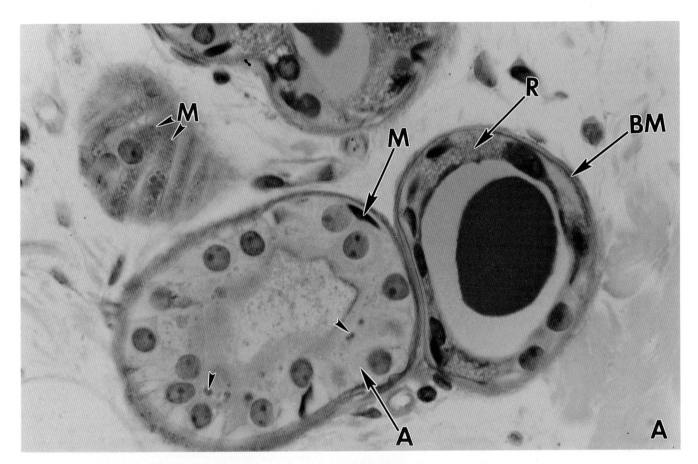

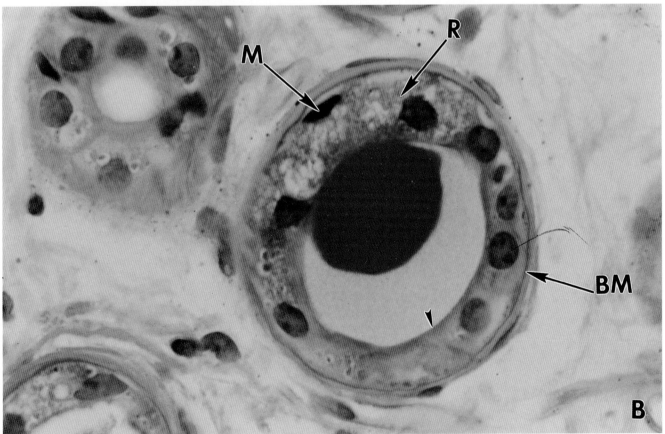

PLATE 131

MIXED GLANDS

Pigment

A. These tubules from the facial skin of a young Black woman are lined with apocrine-like cells that contain typical eccrine sweat gland pigment granules (P). The granules are always more numerous in exposed than in protected skin. The pigment has not been identified. Note the melanophages (M) in the surrounding dermis. 2-μm plastic section. Fontana-Masson silver technique. OM 700x.

B. This tubule from the same gland as in Figure A is lined primarily with eccrine-like, vacuolated, reticulated cells and contains abundant argyrophilic, non-iron-containing pigment typical of eccrine sweat glands. The luminal content is mostly debris of discarded cells including pigment granules. 2-μm plastic section. Fontana-Masson silver technique. OM 700x.

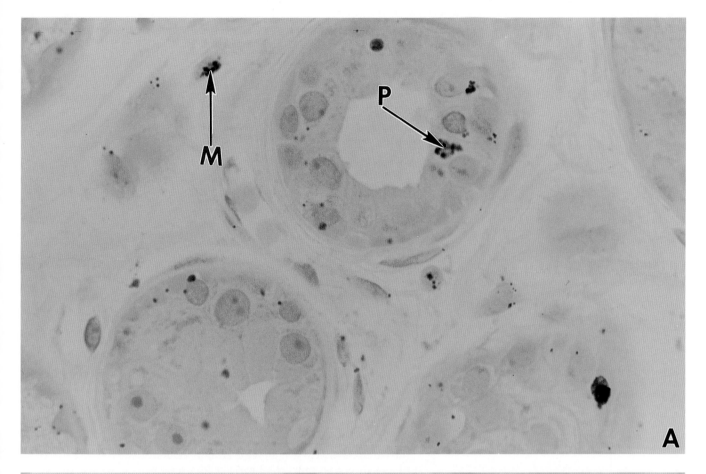

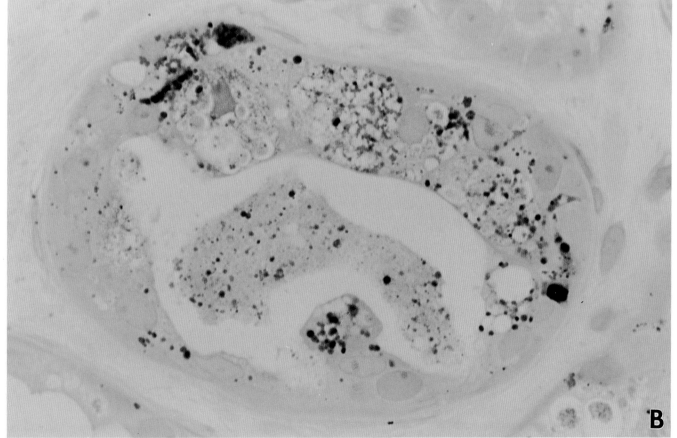

PLATE 132

BUCCAL GLANDS

Ancillary Salivary Glands

Buccal Mucosa

The inside of the cheeks and lips is peppered with many mucoid and some serous ancillary salivary glands. These glands can be felt with the tongue as scattered, pebbly elevations under the buccal and oral mucosa.

A. Mucoid glands (M) inside the lower lip of a 72-year-old man; there are no serous glands. Note the duct (D) and the many large, dark-stained plasma cells (arrowheads) in the connective tissue interstices. Plasma cells are encountered often in apparently normal human tissues. 2-μm plastic section. H and Lee. OM 160x.

B. The secretory cells of these mucoid glands inside the lower lip of the same 72-year-old man stain a light pink color. Note the dark-blue-staining plasma cells (arrowheads) scattered in the connective tissue interstices. 2-μm plastic section. Giemsa stain. OM 250x.

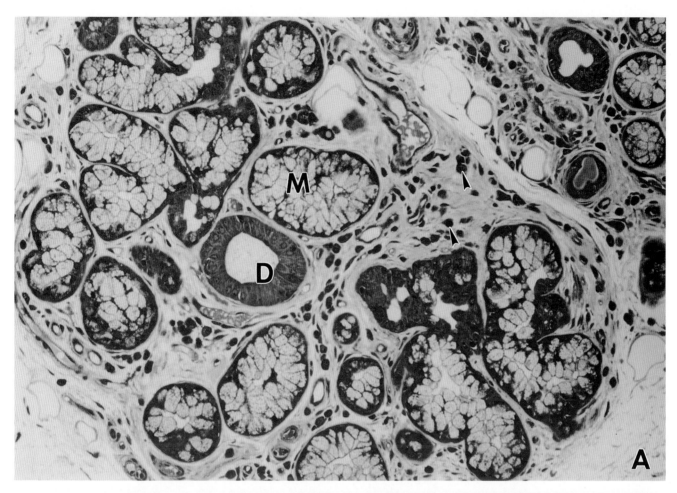

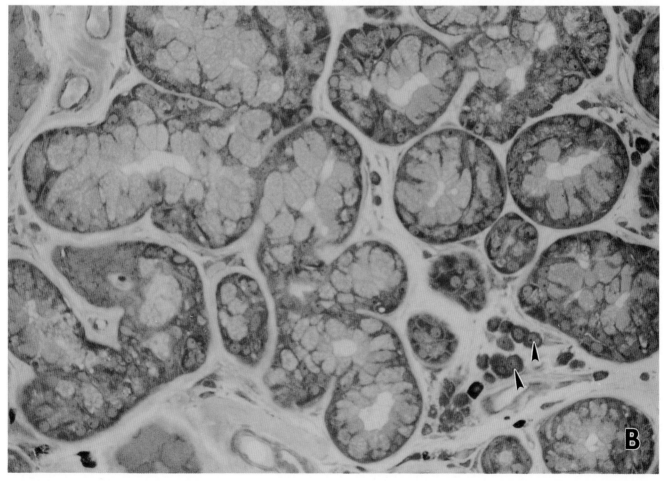

PLATE 133

BUCCAL GLANDS

Ancillary Salivary Glands

Buccal Mucosa

A. These glandular tubules are lined with mucous cells that are mostly laden with strongly PAS-reactive lobules. From inside the lip of a 72-year-old man. 4-μm plastic section. PAS. OM 400x.

B. The mucous globules inside the secretory cells also stain with Hale's colloidal iron technique for mucoproteins. From inside the lip of a 72-year-old man. 4-μm plastic section. Hale's colloidal iron technique, pH 3.0, counterstained with nuclear fast red. OM 250x.

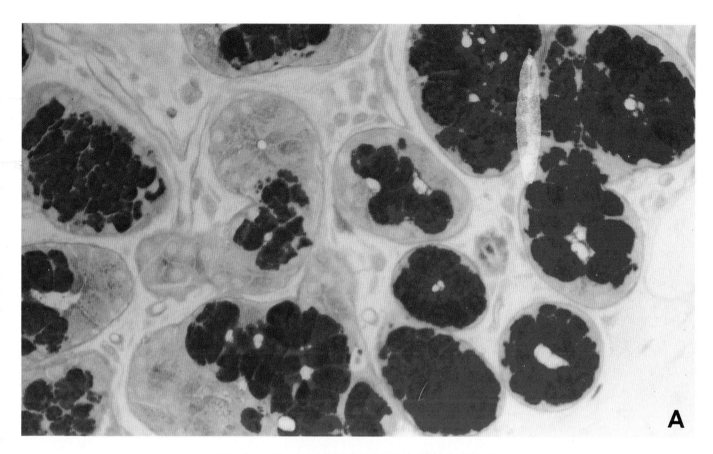

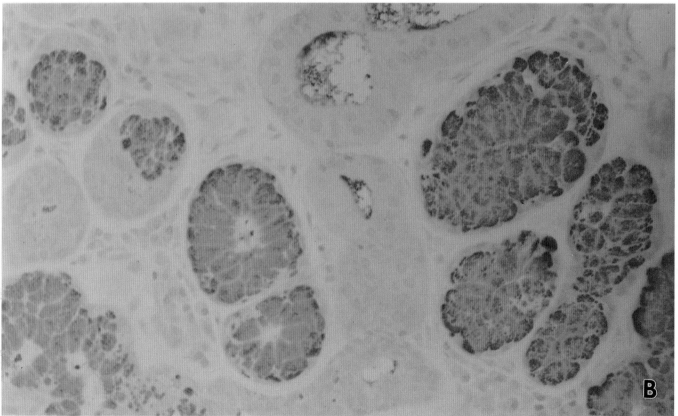

PLATE 134

SEBACEOUS GLANDS

Structure

Human skin has many sebaceous glands, which vary from the single-celled glands of Wolff in the epidermis of the eyelids to the gigantic sebaceous follicles of the face. Sebaceous glands are found in all areas of the skin except the palms, the soles, the digits, and the dorsum of the feet. The glands are largest in the head and around the anogenital orifices. Short ducts connect the large, multiacinar glands to the main duct, and each gland is usually associated with a hair follicle. When very large, the glands are called sebaceous follicles, which open onto the skin through a visible pilosebaceous orifice. When not accompanied by a hair follicle, they are referred to as free sebaceous glands. These glands are found in the vermilion border of the lips, the mucous membranes of the buccal and oral cavities, the labia minora, the nipple of the breast, and the inside of the eyelids. Sebaceous glands are small in childhood and enlarge at puberty. The free glands on the buccal and oral mucous membranes become more numerous and larger in both men and women after the age of 40. These oddly located sebaceous glands are not usually associated with hair follicles, and their ducts open directly onto the surface of the mucosa.

A. Sebaceous glands, like hair, are unique to the skin of mammals. Their size and structure vary from area to area. They may be unilobular or multiacinar. The structural plan of most multiacinar sebaceous glands resembles that of a cauliflower. Notwithstanding the size and numbers of sebaceous glands, there is little known about the biological significance of sebum.

B. Rosettes of free sebaceous glands in the mouth (Fordyce spots) of a 60-year-old woman, stained whole with the lipophilic dye Sudan IV. OM 15x. Courtesy of Prof. A. E. W. Miles.

C. Sebaceous glands in the gingiva of the same 60-year-old woman. Thick frozen section stained with Sudan IV and counterstained with hematoxylin. OM 10x. Courtesy of Prof. A. E. W. Miles.

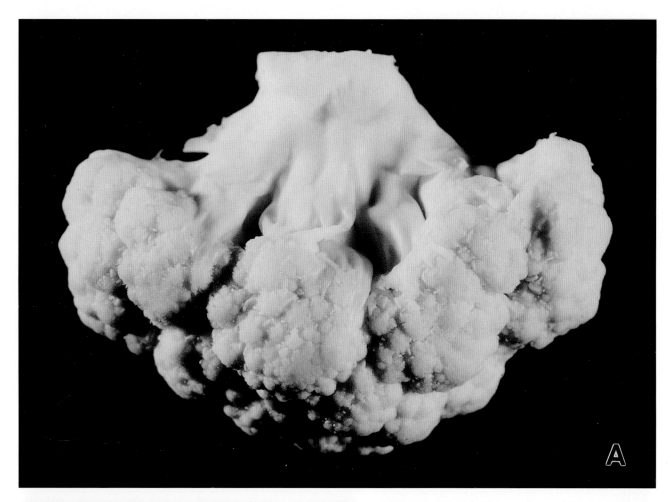

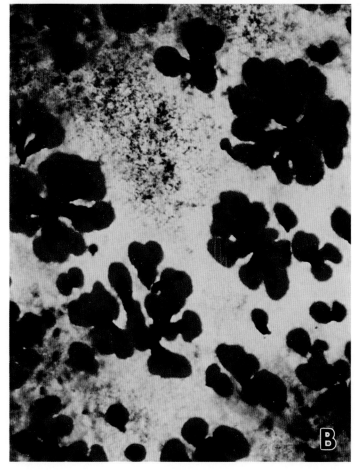

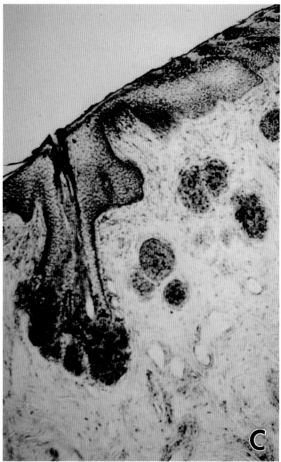

PLATE 135

SEBACEOUS GLANDS
Fetus

Sebaceous glands are large at birth and are the first exocrine glands to mature in the fetus. They are very sensitive to androgenic stimulation. In the fetus they are under the influence of maternal androgens. The glands atrophy after birth and remain small in children until early puberty, when they are stimulated by endogenous androgens. This results in maturation and enlargement of the glands.

A. Large, cauliflower-like sebaceous glands on the outer cutaneous surface of the lip of an 8-month female fetus, encircled by many branching blood vessels. 40-μm frozen section. Gomori's alkaline phosphatase technique. OM 100x.

B. Sebaceous follicle from an ala of the nose of an 8-month fetus with an enlarged pilosebaceous canal (P). The "empty" canal was probably filled with keratinous material. Sebum, the product of sebaceous glands, contributes to the vernix caseosa during fetal life. Note the lanugo hair follicles (arrows). 40-μm frozen section. Gomori's alkaline phosphatase technique. OM 100x.

C. Sebaceous follicle from an ala of the nose of an 8-month fetus. The dilated pilosebaceous canal (P) is full of sloughed horny cells in a matrix of sebum. 40-μm frozen section. Roman's AOV elastic fiber technique. OM 100x.

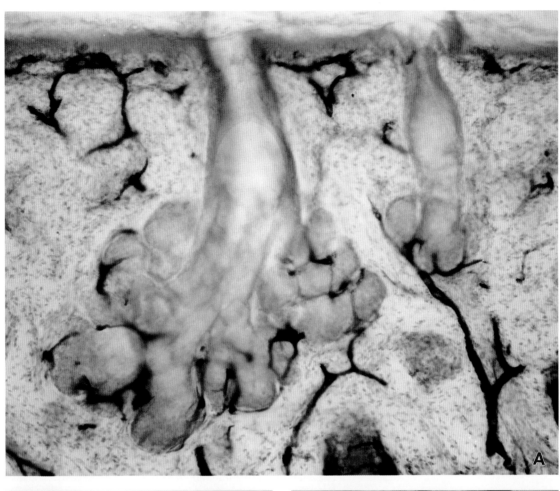

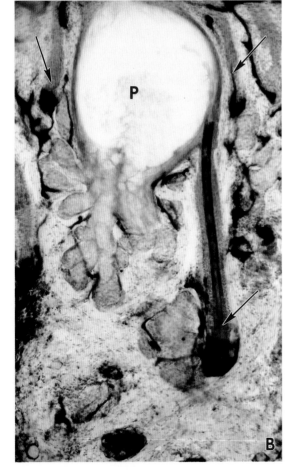

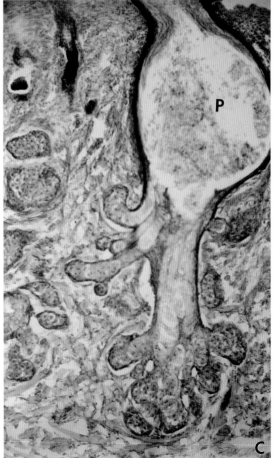

PLATE 136

SEBACEOUS GLANDS

Face, Scalp

The largest sebaceous glands are usually found on the face, scalp, and genitalia. They are associated with hair follicles and empty through a duct into the follicular canal.

A. Sebaceous glands open into the pilary canal of a scalp hair follicle of a 17-year-old man. Note the long arrector pili muscle (AP), which forms a sling that cradles the sebaceous gland. 6-μm paraffin section. H and E. OM 100x. Courtesy of Prof. Antonio Tosti.

B. Sebaceous gland opening into the pilary canal of a terminal hair follicle from the scalp of a young woman. The inner root sheath (IRS) and its corrugations (C) line the pilary canal just below the entrance of the sebaceous duct (D). The smaller sebaceous gland (*) is attached to a vellus hair follicle (V). 2-μm plastic section. H and Lee. OM 100x.

C. In this sebaceous follicle from the face, undifferentiated cells (arrows) are at the periphery, and some are scattered throughout the acinus. Lipid differentiation generally proceeds in a centripetal direction. These large lobules abut against a large arrector pili muscle (AP). 2-μm plastic section. H and Lee. OM 250x.

D. Vellus hair follicle from the photodamaged face of a 36-year-old woman. The sebaceous glands have largely disappeared; all that remains are undifferentiated anlagen (A). Remnants of sebaceous glands are usually found in sun-damaged skin and in the skin of old people. Note the sun-damaged elastic tissue (E) in the upper dermis. 2-μm plastic section. H and Lee. OM 160x.

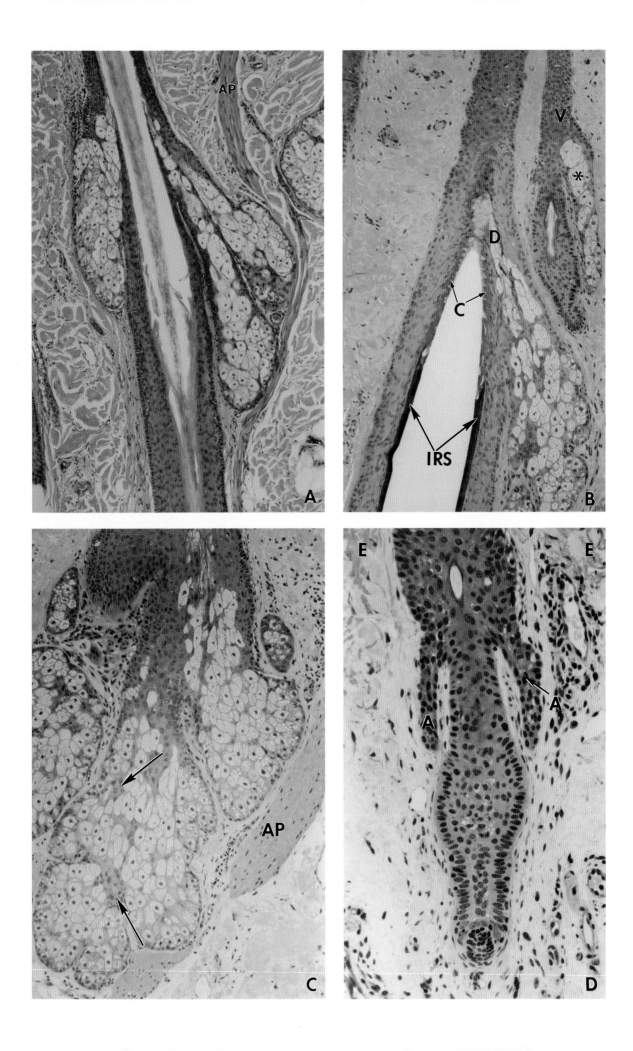

PLATE 137

SEBACEOUS GLANDS

Face

A. In this sebaceous follicle from the face of a 35-year-old woman, the anagen vellus hair follicle is an appendage of the large, multi-lobulated gland. The club of the vellus hair (CH) is still anchored in the cell capsule. Dermal papilla (P). Blood vessel (BV). The new follicle is in early anagen (HG). 2-μm plastic section. H and Lee. OM 100x.

B. Large sebaceous gland acinus surrounded by a basement membrane (BM) and a thick collagenous capsule (C). The cells at the periphery of the acinus are undifferentiated (UC). 2-μm plastic section. H and Lee. OM 400x.

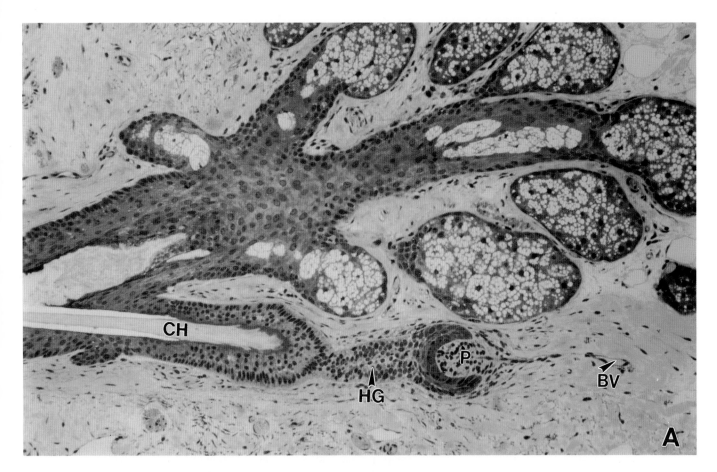

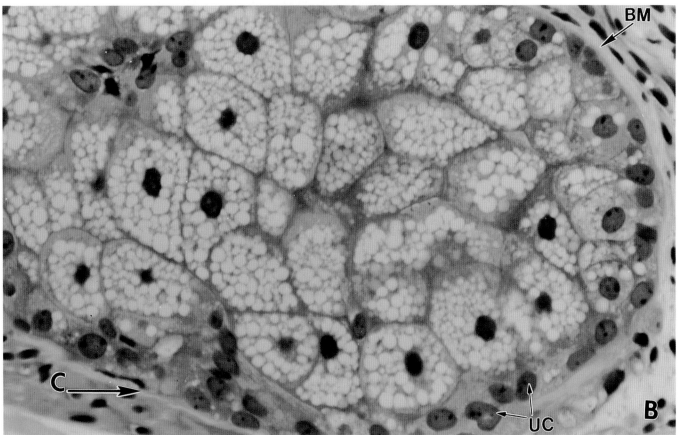

PLATE 138

SEBACEOUS GLANDS

Maturation of Sebaceous Glands

A. The cells at the periphery of this sebaceous acinus are just beginning to differentiate by forming lipid globules in their cytoplasm. Sebum vesicles are first synthesized in the Golgi body near the nucleus. As the cells attain maturity, they acquire a foamy appearance and may enlarge in volume by more than 100-fold. Some sebaceous acini are anchored to the dermis by fine elastic fibers (arrows). Artery (At). 4-μm plastic section. Verhoff's hematoxylin. OM 630x.

B. Mature sebaceous cells near the center of an acinus. Each cell contains both small and large lipid globules. Some large globules are composed of coalescing, smaller fatty vesicles. The lipid vesicles are surrounded by dark-staining material (arrows), which has been shown to contain mitochondria. 4-μm plastic section. Verhoff's hematoxylin. OM 630x.

C. Sebaceous glands exhibit holocrine secretion. The nuclei and all of the cytoplasmic components of mature cells become distorted and may disappear. In this photograph of the duct (Dt) of a sebaceous gland, the cells disintegrate (CD), rupture, and release lipid, cellular remnants, and keratinous protein (K); this melange is the sebum (Se) released onto the skin surface. Other than its odor, which contributes to the characteristic human scent, the function of sebum is still unknown. 4-μm plastic section. Verhoff's hematoxylin. OM 630x.

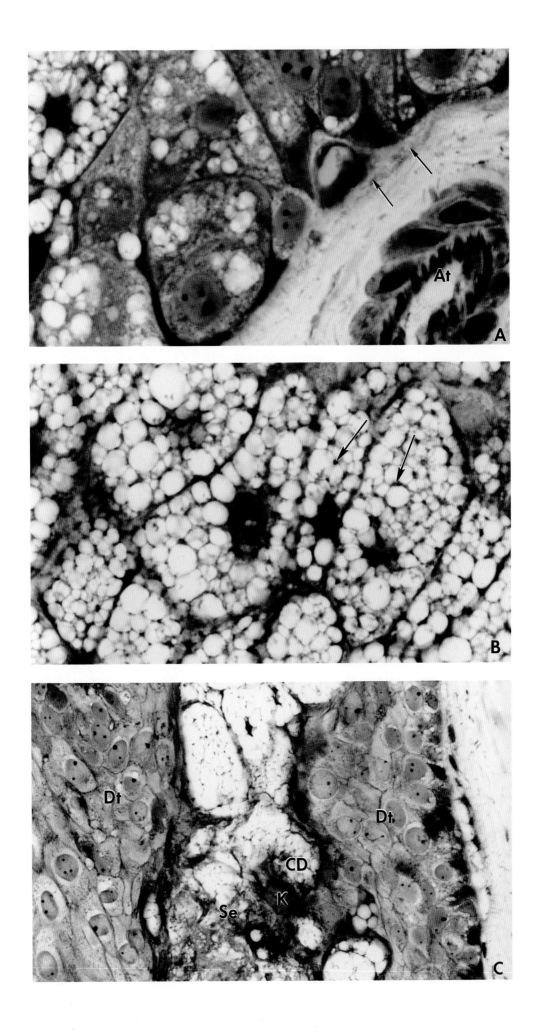

PLATE 139

SEBACEOUS GLANDS

Differentiation

Since sebaceous glands are holocrine, the formation of sebum is dependent upon existing cells and cell proliferation. A mitotic cell (M) in late telophase is at the periphery of an acinus. Differentiating cells are packed with large and small lipid vesicles. Note the undifferentiated cells (UC). 2-μm plastic section. H and Lee. OM 1100x.

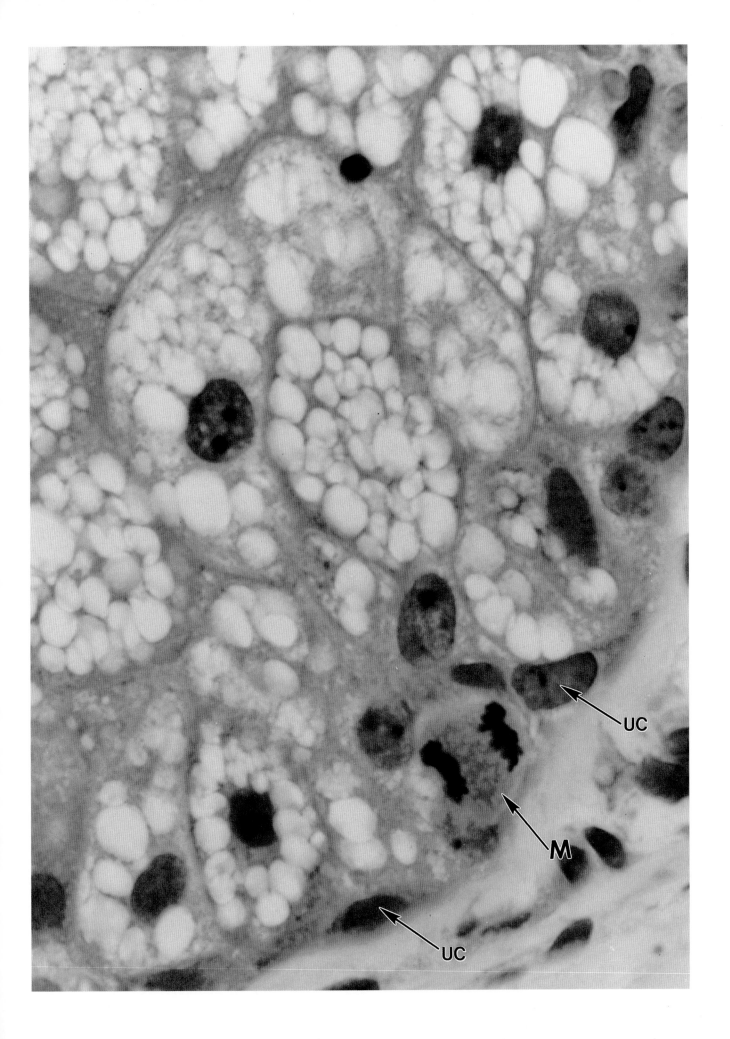

PLATE 140

SEBACEOUS GLANDS
PAS

A. Sebaceous gland acinus surrounded by a PAS-reactive basement membrane (BM). On the outside of the acinus is a thick collagenous capsule. The undifferentiated cells (arrows) at the periphery are full of glycogen granules. Glycogen is distributed inversely to the state of cell differentiation. Histochemically demonstrable glycogen in sebaceous glands is a peculiarity of human skin. 4-μm plastic section. PAS. OM 250x.

B. Enlarged detail of peripheral, undifferentiated sebaceous cells (arrows) with prominent, red, PAS-reactive granules (glycogen). Glycogen decreases as the cells differentiate. Blood vessels (V) lie just outside the basement membrane (BM). 4-μm plastic section. PAS. OM 1200x.

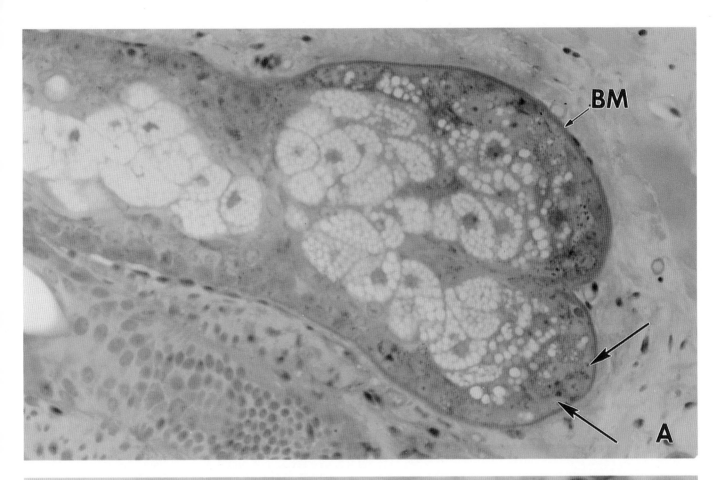

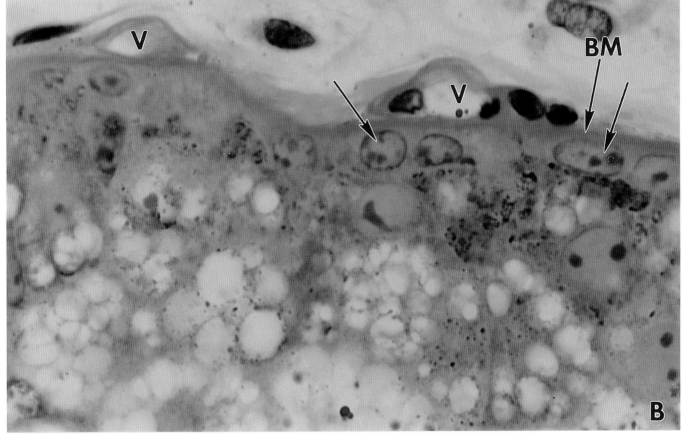

PLATE 141

SEBACEOUS GLANDS

Labia and Nose

A. Sebaceous glands (arrows) attached to a hair follicle from the underside of the epidermis of the mons veneris of a 20-year-old woman. Split-skin preparation. OM 50x.

B. The labia minora of women are studded with large sebaceous glands. This split-skin preparation shows the characteristic swirling pattern of the underside of the epidermis and the large sebaceous glands (arrows). Hair follicles in the labia disappear during late gestation, and the glands are mostly free of hair follicles in women. Sebum is abundantly secreted over the surface of the genitalia and may be responsible for their characteristic odor. OM 50x.

C. Unstained free sebaceous gland with its long, narrow duct (arrow) from the labia minora of a young woman. Split-skin preparation. OM 50x.

D. The skin of the nose is a solid bed of sebaceous glands. These gigantic sebaceous follicles from the ala of the nose of a young man are associated with vellus hair follicles (VHF). 8-μm paraffin section. H and E. OM 120x.

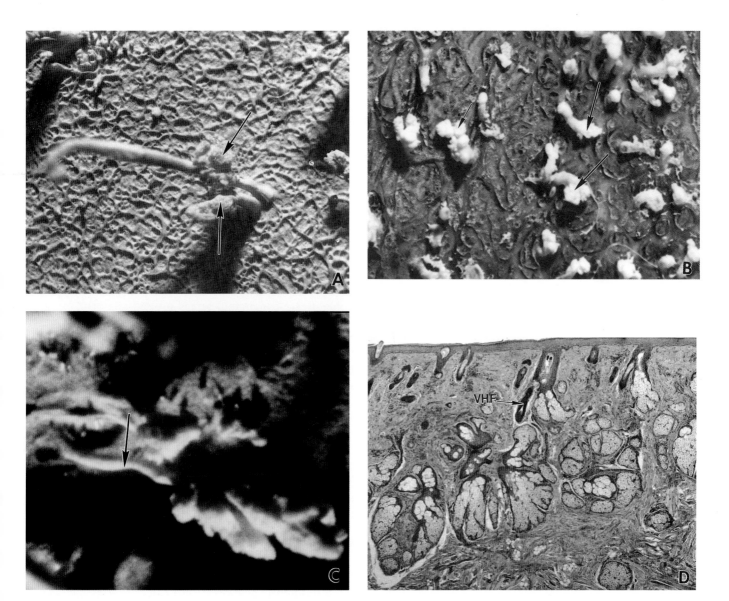

PLATE 142

SEBACEOUS GLANDS

A. The rich blood supply (black) of a large sebaceous gland in the earlobe of a young man attests to the high energy requirements of these glands. Acini (Ac). Duct (Dt). 20-μm frozen section. Gomori's alkaline phosphatase technique. OM 120x.

B. Acetylcholinesterase-containing nerves around the acini of a meibomian gland (Mb) in the eyelid of a 21-year-old man. These are the largest free sebaceous glands in the body. Skeins of fine, non-myelinated nerve fibers are wrapped around the glands. The nerves around meibomian glands probably function as sensory receptors. 20-μm frozen section. Koelle's acetylcholinesterase technique. OM 120x.

C. Melanocytes are numerous on the surface of this large sebaceous gland in the nipple of a 23-year-old White woman. Sebaceous glands in the labia minora of young women also contain estrogen-sensitive melanocytes. Melanocytes have not been seen in the glands of the breast and genitalia of old women. 20-μm frozen section. Winkelmann's silver impregnation method. OM 120x.

D. Contact photomicrograph of sebaceous glands in the face of a 50-year-old man. A 5-μm unstained paraffin section was placed next to a photosensitive film, which was exposed to ultraviolet light, 2580 nm, and the film was developed. Most of the ultraviolet absorption (lighter portions) occurred in the nuclei, connective tissue, and vellus hair follicle (H). The lipid droplets had no ultraviolet absorption. OM 250x. Courtesy of Prof. Antonio Tosti.

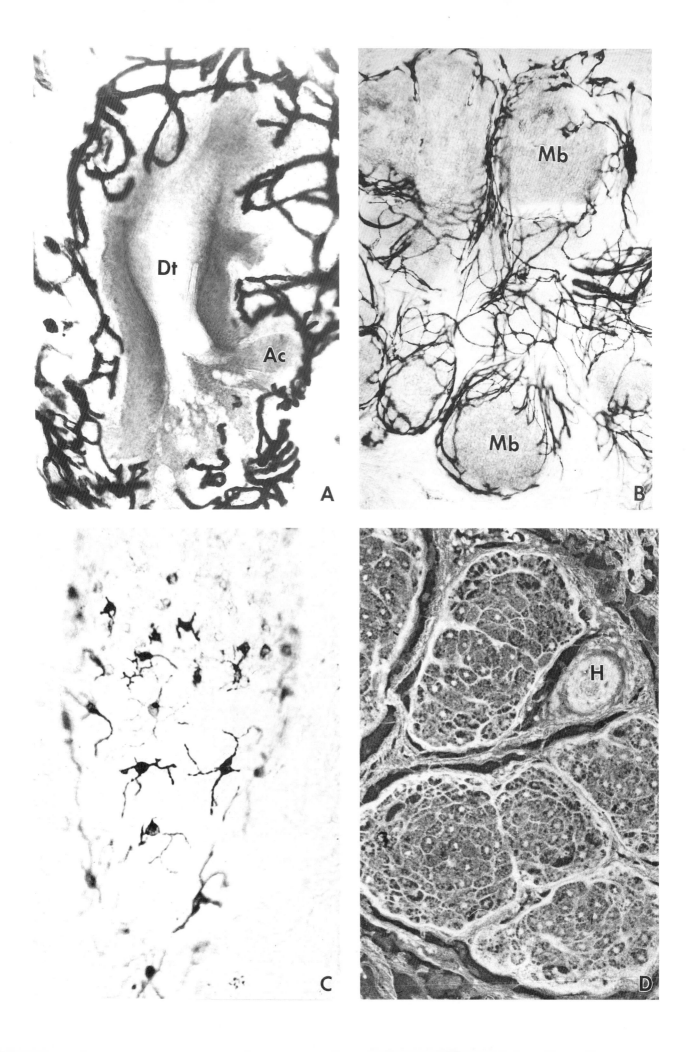

PLATE 143

SEBACEOUS GLANDS
Cryofractured

A. SEM micrograph of lyophilized, cryofractured facial skin of an adolescent young man, with two emerging hairs (arrows) surrounded by abundant sebaceous tissue (S). OM 500x. Courtesy of Dr. Dennis D. Knutson.

B. SEM micrograph of many sebaceous gland fragments (S) near a hair follicle. Sebaceous tissue also abuts against the connective tissue layer (Ct) of the hair follicle. OM 500x. Courtesy of Dr. Dennis D. Knutson.

C. SEM micrograph of a sebaceous gland acinus surrounded by connective tissue (Ct). The individual cell boundaries can be seen well toward the center of the acinus. Each cell is like a bag of large and small marbles, the "marbles" corresponding to the lipid globules. OM 600x. Reprinted by permission of VCH Publishers, Inc., 220 East 23rd St., New York, N.Y. 10010 from Wilborn, Hyde and Montes, *SEM of Normal and Abnormal Human Skin*, p. 102, 1985.

D. Highly magnified SEM micrograph of sebaceous cells in the facial skin of an adolescent young man, showing only a few cells and the connective tissue (Ct) between them. Each compartment in this photograph is a single cell full of fat globules. OM 6000x. Courtesy of Dr. Dennis D. Knutson.

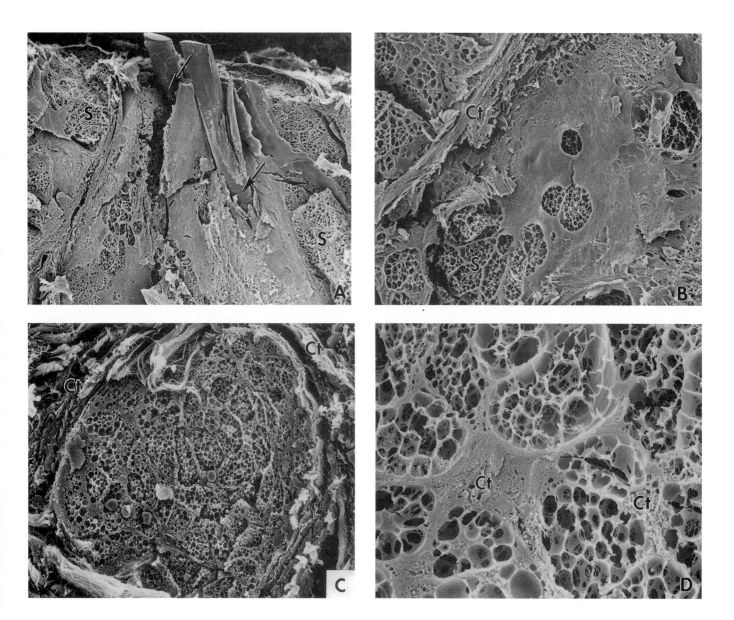

Hair and Hair Follicles

It is fashionable to refer to man as a naked ape, meaning a hairless ape. This witty designation, however, is completely wrong, since we are certainly not hairless and we are not apes. We are abundantly supplied with hairs, but most of them are barely visible to the naked eye. Quantitatively, we probably have as many hairs in our skin as furry animals.

PLATE 144

VELLUS and TERMINAL HAIRS

Hairs are complex keratinous cylinders packed inside a tight girdle of imbricated cortical scales. Hairs can be divided into (1) vellus hairs, which are fine, unmedullated, soft, unpigmented, and relatively short, and (2) terminal hairs, which are coarser, longer, and mostly pigmented and medullated. There are also intermediate hairs. All fetal hairs are called lanugo hairs.

A. SEM micrograph of the surface of the tragus of an old man. Vellus hairs (V) of different sizes, some difficult to see with the naked eye, grow between coarse, intermediate, or terminal (T) hairs. OM 120x.

B. SEM micrograph of the surface of a knee of an old man. A number of vellus hairs emerge in tufts (V). Note the imprints left on the surface by terminal (T) or intermediate hairs that were compressed against the skin (arrows). The surface of old skin is crisscrossed by many lines. OM 120x.

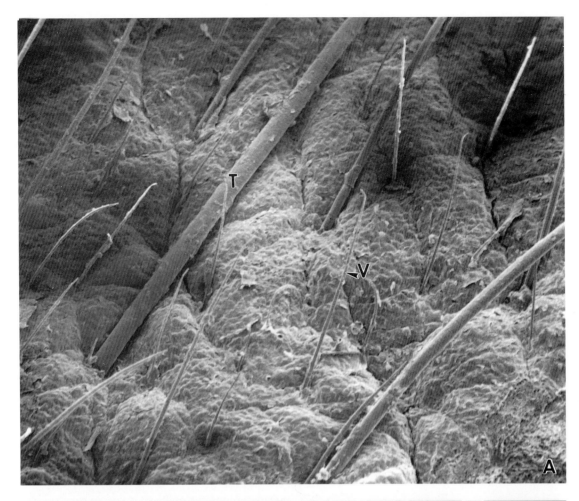

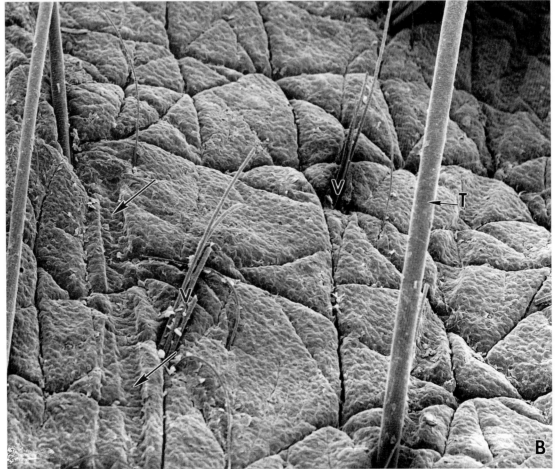

PLATE 145

VELLUS and
TERMINAL HAIRS

Hairs are found nearly everywhere on the body. The only glabrous skin is on the palms and soles, the dorsal skin of the last phalanges of the digits, the glans penis, the clitoris, and the vermilion border of the lips.

At puberty, under the influence of androgens, some vellus hairs are replaced by terminal hairs in the pubic area and the axilla in both men and women. Body hairs continue to change in men after puberty. The type of hair can change, but not the number of hairs.

A. SEM micrograph of a terminal chest hair of a middle-aged White man. The thickness of body hairs increases with age. About 90% of men's chest hairs consist of terminal and intermediate hairs, but fewer than 35% of women's body hairs are terminal or intermediate. OM 200x. Courtesy of Dr. P. Goodkin.

B. SEM micrograph of the axilla of a young woman, showing two terminal hairs (T) emerging from one orifice, and a vellus hair (V). The hairs in the axilla participate in the dispersal of axillary odors. OM 200x. Courtesy of Dr. P. Goodkin.

C. SEM micrograph of the convoluted surface of the elbow of an old man. Vellus hairs (arrows) emerge between the convolutions. OM 40x. Courtesy of Dr. P. Goodkin.

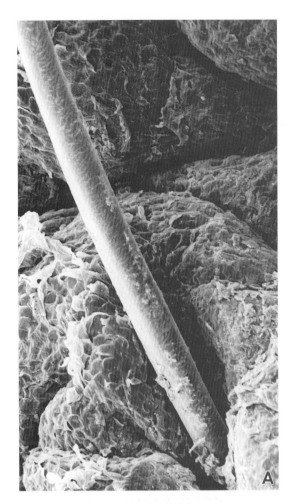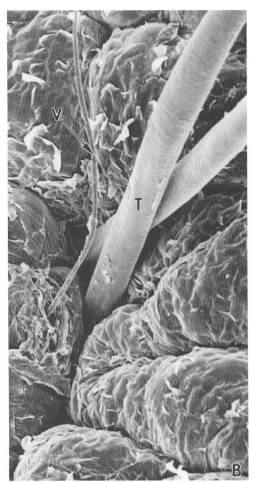

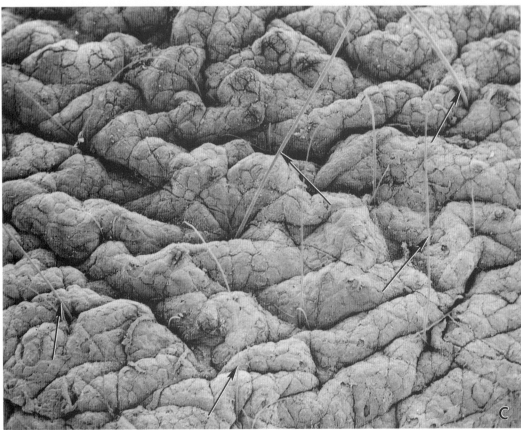

PLATE 146

HAIRS

Each hair follicle, the principal epidermal appendage, produces a unique hair that is not identical with any other hair. A new follicle generates each subsequent hair in the growth cycles that follow.

A. SEM micrograph of the surface of the nose of a young man. A short vellus hair emerges through the orifice of a sebaceous follicle, which is filled with horny debris. OM 200x. Courtesy of Dr. P. Goodkin.

B. SEM micrograph of the dermal surface of skin from the thigh of a young woman, showing a bundle of intermediate hairs. The inner root sheath (IRS) envelops this bundle of hairs (arrow). Farther down in the dermis or hypodermis, each of these hairs probably had an individual follicle. Hairs often merge to become adjacent near the surface. A vellus hair (V) is nearby. Connective tissue sheath (CT). Cryofracture. OM 120x.

C. Surface of the nape of an old man with tufts of hairs emerging from single orifices. Many of these hairs have an intermediate size (IH); some are obviously vellus hairs (V). Note the surface markings characteristic of old skin. OM 40x. Courtesy of Dr. P. Goodkin.

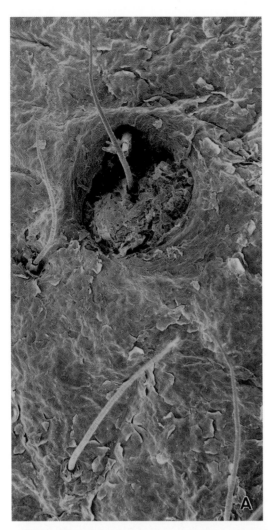
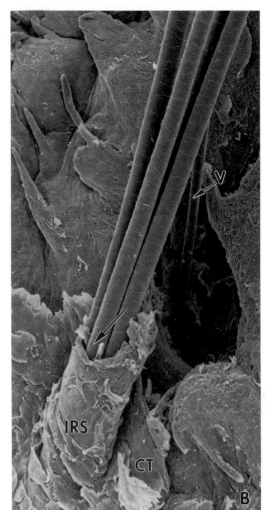
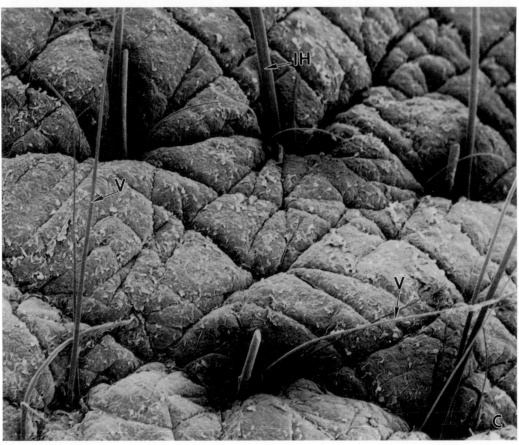

PLATE 147

HAIR SHAFT

In contrast to those in other regions, the follicles in the scalp can grow continuously for years and produce very long hairs. (These long hairs are said to protect the head from solar radiation.) The major portion of the hair shaft is the cortex, which is surrounded by a cuticle with its free margins directed toward the tip of the hair. The cuticle scales, which are arranged like overlapping tiles on a roof, are translucent and mostly nonpigmented.

The following photographs are SEM views of different levels of a 12-inch-long scalp hair. Courtesy of Dr. W. H. Fahrenbach.

A. The split end of the 12-inch-long hair. The cuticle is mostly worn off, exposing the cortex, which is clearly falling apart. OM 500x.

B. The hair about 6 inches above its base. The cuticle cells are frayed and broken, perhaps as a result of combing and/or brushing. OM 500x.

C. The base of the scalp hair as it emerges from the orifice. The imbricated cuticle consists of smooth-edged cells that bind and protect the cortex. OM 500x.

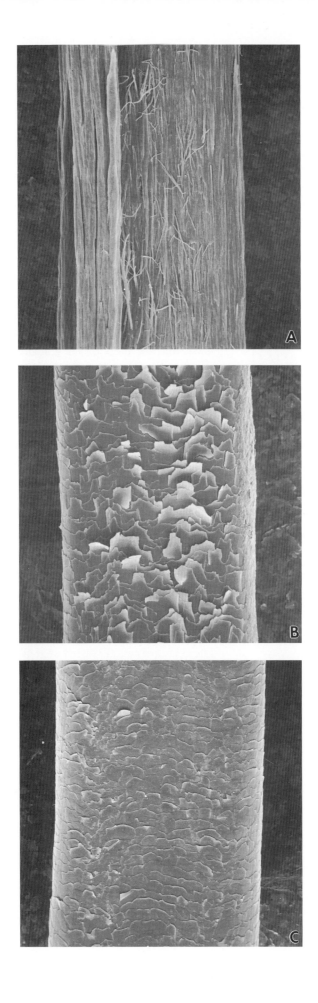

PLATE 148

EYELASHES

Human beings and the hairless whales are the only mammals that have no vibrissae or sinus hairs; even the great apes have vibrissae. Coarse vibrissa hairs grow from highly innervated and vascularized follicles. Some investigators believe that the supracilia (eyebrow hairs) and the hairs of the glabella (the space above the bridge of the nose between the eyebrows) are all that remains of vibrissae in human beings. There is some merit to such a belief, because the follicles of these hairs are exceedingly well vascularized and innervated.

Eyelashes and eyebrows in human beings protect the eyes from solar radiation and from foreign particles. Eyebrows are also used with facial expressions. The follicles of these hairs are generously supplied with nerves.

A. Thick frozen section through the tarsal plate of an eyelid of an old man. A meibomian gland (MG) and its duct (arrow) are prominent above the cilia follicles (C). The cilia (eyelashes) have typical hair follicles with small sebaceous glands called tarsal glands (T). Note that the bulb of the cilium follicle does not reside within a fatty bed. Elastic fibers are sparse in the eyelid. 40-μm frozen section. Roman's AOV elastic fiber technique. OM 120x.

B. Horizontal section through the palpebral border of an old man. The cilia (arrows) are distributed in such a way that any two or three adjacent ones could be shed without forming a substantial gap. 40-μm frozen section. Hematoxylin. OM 50x.

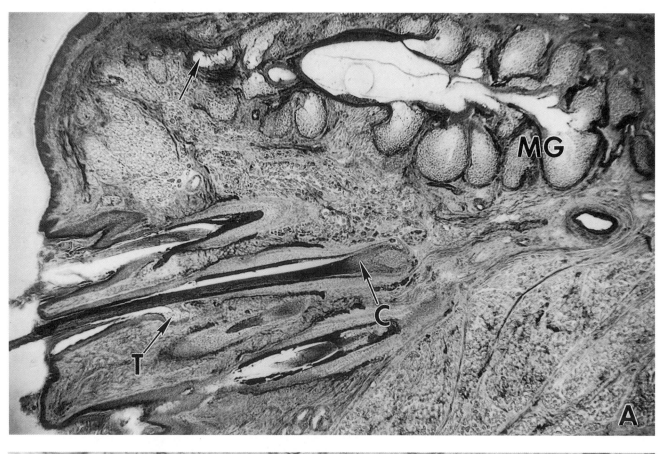

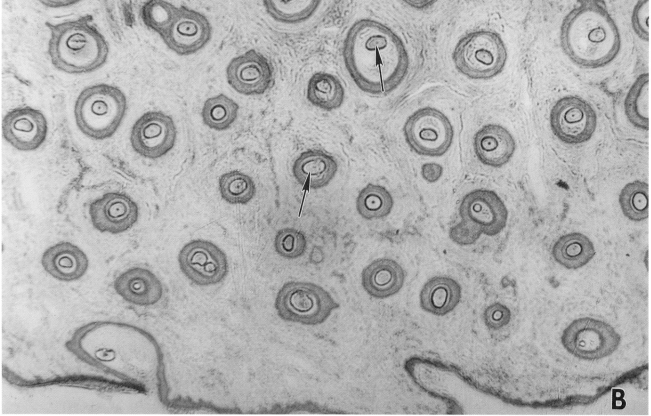

PLATE 149

HAIRS

Ears

Even though one does not usually think of the ears, and particularly those of women, as being hairy, ears have many hair follicles in both men and women.

A. Many hair follicles in the ear of an 8-month fetal girl. Development of general body hair in the fetus starts during the fourth month. Split-skin preparation. OM 120x.

B. In the ear of a 72-year-old woman, the hair follicles are large and widely separated. Split-skin preparation. OM 120x.

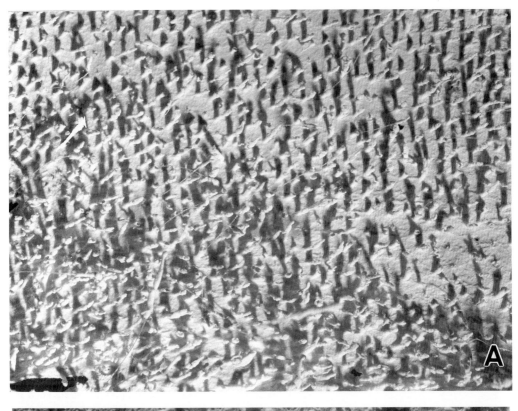

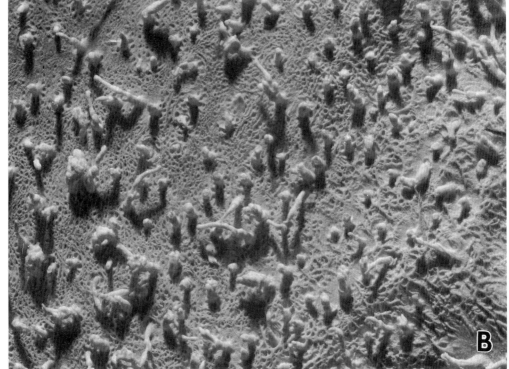

PLATE 150

UNDERSURFACE of FETAL SCALP

During the second and third fetal months, the first cutaneous appendages appear as primordial hair follicles in the eyebrows, upper lip, and chin; these are regions that bear vibrissae in other mammals. Follicles continue to develop asynchronously during the fourth month and for the remainder of fetal life. When first formed, all follicles produce lanugo hairs that resemble postnatal vellus hairs. As the skin expands, additional primary follicles are formed; secondary follicles are formed alongside them. The hairs are usually in groups of three to five. The density of the hair follicle population decreases as the body surface increases. No one has shown that new follicles can develop in adult skin.

A. Undersurface of the epidermis of the scalp of a 6-month fetus, showing many developing groups of hair follicles. Each group consists of a primary follicle (P) flanked by secondary follicles (arrows). The humps (E) between the follicles are primordial eccrine sweat glands. Split-skin preparation. OM 100x.

B. Primordial hair group from the same fetal scalp as in Figure A. The basal cells of both the epidermis and the outer root sheath of the hair follicles are somewhat polyhedral. This group contains one primary follicle (P) and two secondary follicles (arrows). In the center of the primary hair follicle is the lanugo hair shaft and the inner root sheath. Split-skin preparation. OM 250x.

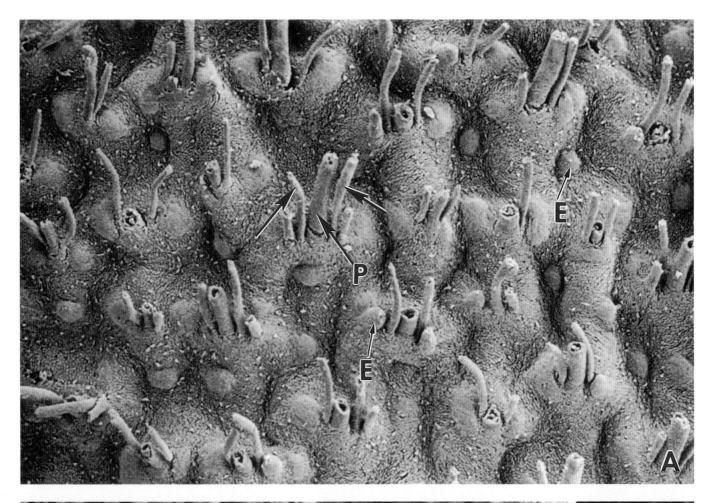

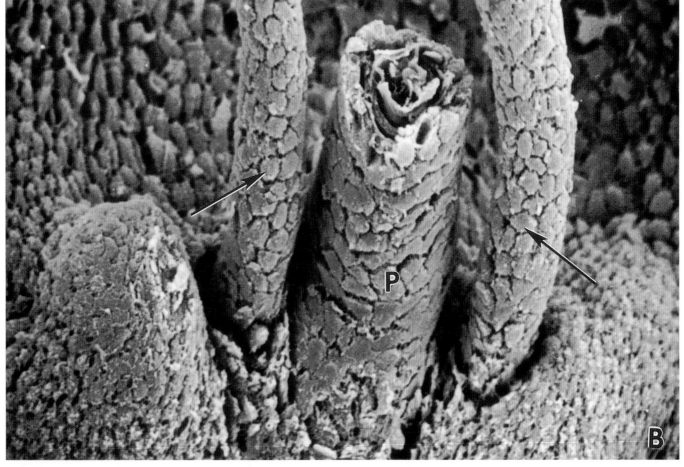

PLATE 151

CRYOFRACTURE of HAIRS

These illustrations of the scalp of a young White man were prepared by cryofracture and photographed with the SEM by Dr. Dennis D. Knutson. OM 1000x.

A. Pilary canal just below the entrance of the sebaceous glands. The hair shaft (H) is shattered but shows the surrounding cuticle cells. Around the hair is the inner root sheath (IR).

B. This pilary canal (PC) and the infundibulum, near the surface, are full of keratinous material. The hair has been lost, but the shaft of a vellus hair (arrowhead) is nearby. The papillary dermis (PD) under the epidermis (E) consists of collagenous fibers smaller than those of the reticular dermis (RD).

C. Surface of a hair midway up the follicle with its intact cuticle cells (C) interlocking with the cuticle cells of the inner root sheath (CI). This arrangement anchors the hair firmly inside the follicle.

D. Each follicle is encased in a well-organized connective tissue sheath (CT) consisting of dense collagen bundles wrapped circularly around the follicle, and an outer layer with the collagen fibers oriented longitudinally. Outside the latter are the thick collagenous fibers (Co) of the reticular dermis.

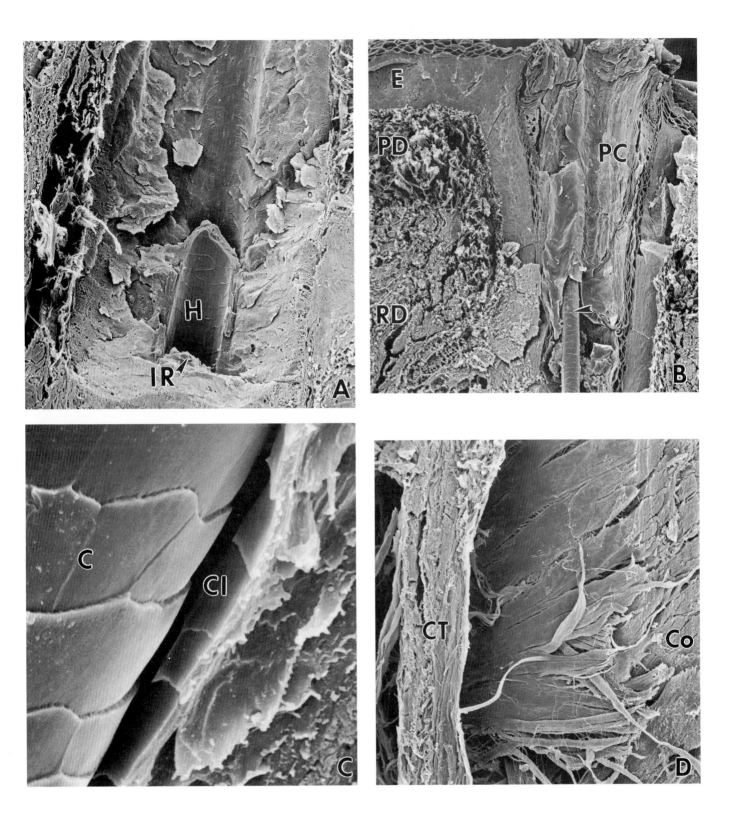

PLATE 152

HAIR FOLLICLES
Scalp

Terminal hair follicle, in the scalp of an 11-year-old boy, with its bulb (B) deep in a papilla adiposa of the hypodermis (Hy). The cut through the center shows the continuous medulla (M) in the hair shaft. Terminal hairs of adolescent boys vary from 30 to 80 μm in diameter. A smaller intermediate hair (SH) is accompanied by a vellus follicle (V). The blood vessels are stained black with the alkaline phosphatase technique. Hair follicles are vascularized primarily around the bulb and the upper part, or infundibulum (I). Sebaceous glands (S) open into the infundibulum of the follicle. Eccrine sweat glands (E) are richly vascularized. 40-μm frozen section. Gomori's alkaline phosphatase technique. OM 125x.

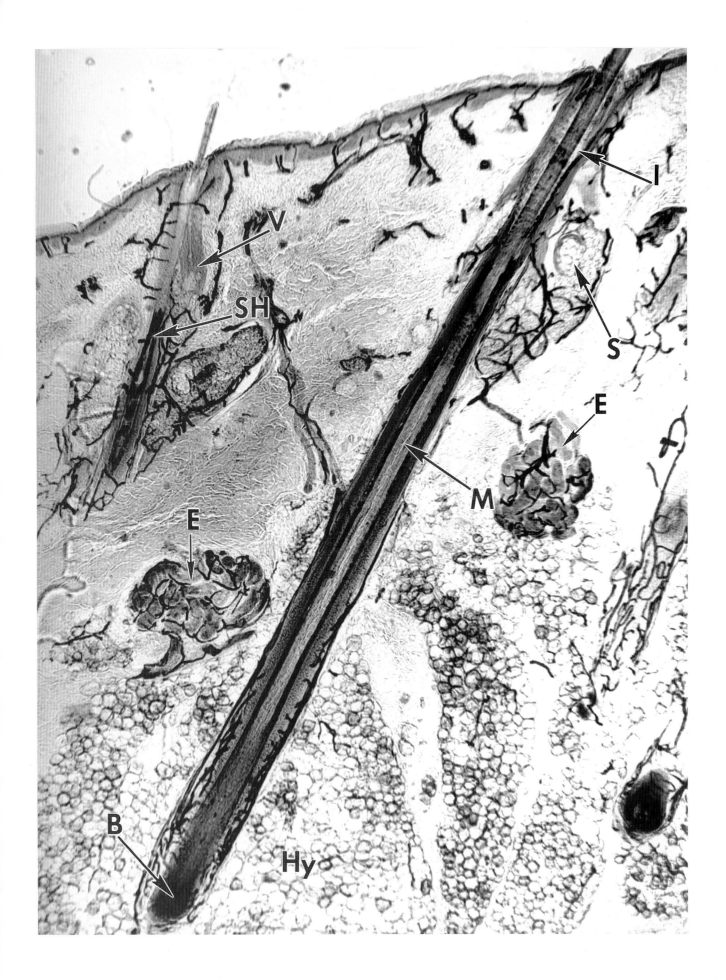

PLATE 153

DIAGRAM of an ANAGEN FOLLICLE

The anagen follicle is divided into a permanent upper end and a transient lower portion lying below the bulge. The bulge is a bump on the follicle's outer root sheath into which the arrector pili inserts. At the end of the period of growth (anagen), the follicle undergoes a complex involution known as catagen. During the catagen phase, all of the "transient" portions of the follicle degenerate.

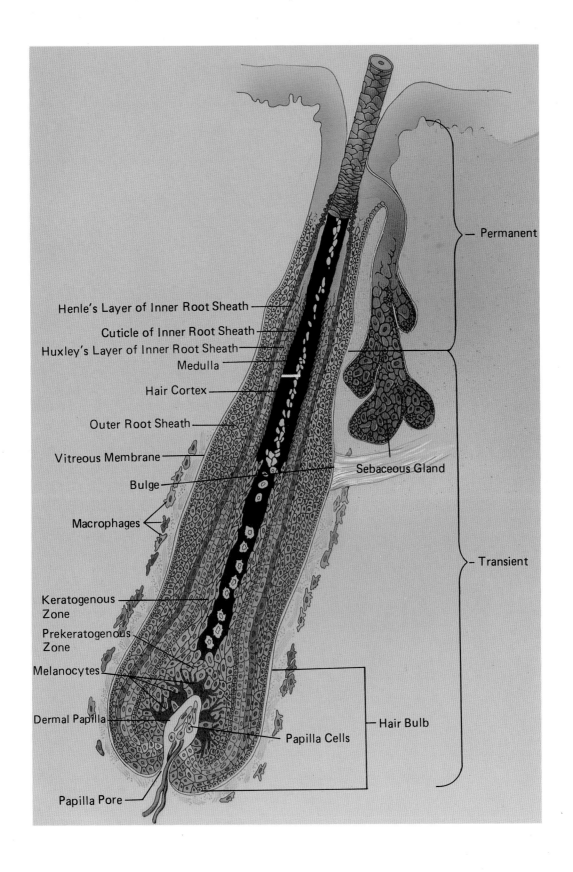

Henle's Layer of Inner Root Sheath

Cuticle of Inner Root Sheath

Huxley's Layer of Inner Root Sheath

Medulla

Hair Cortex

Outer Root Sheath

Vitreous Membrane

Bulge

Macrophages

Keratogenous Zone

Prekeratogenous Zone

Melanocytes

Dermal Papilla

Papilla Pore

Permanent

Sebaceous Gland

Transient

Hair Bulb

Papilla Cells

PLATE 154

ANAGEN HAIR FOLLICLE

Lower part of a terminal hair follicle in anagen, from the scalp of a young White man. Undifferentiated matrix cells (Ma) are aligned in rows as they ascend from the matrix of the bulb (B) to the keratogenous zone (K). The matrix cells give rise to all the cells of the hair follicle: the hair shaft (medulla, cortex, and cuticle) the inner root sheath [Henle's layer (he), Huxley's layer (hx), and the cuticle of the inner root sheath (cir)], and the outer root sheath (ORS). Henle's layer is the first element to become cornified, just above the bulb. The cuticle cells (CC) of the hair shaft begin to be keratinized at about the same level as Henle's layer.

In the center of the hair cortex (Co) is the interrupted row of medulla cells (M). Melanocytes (Mc) are situated over the papilla and give the hair its color. The dermal papilla (P) is cut through its center. Spindle cells (sp) separate potential inner root sheath (IRS) cells from potential outer root sheath cells. The basement membrane lies between the outer root sheath and the glassy or vitreous membrane (V). Outside the vitreous membrane is a two-layered connective tissue sheath (CT). The inner, or circular, layer is wrapped around the follicle; the outer, or longitudinal, layer runs along the follicle. These layers converge and fuse just below the dermal papilla. 2-μm plastic section. H and Lee. OM 250x.

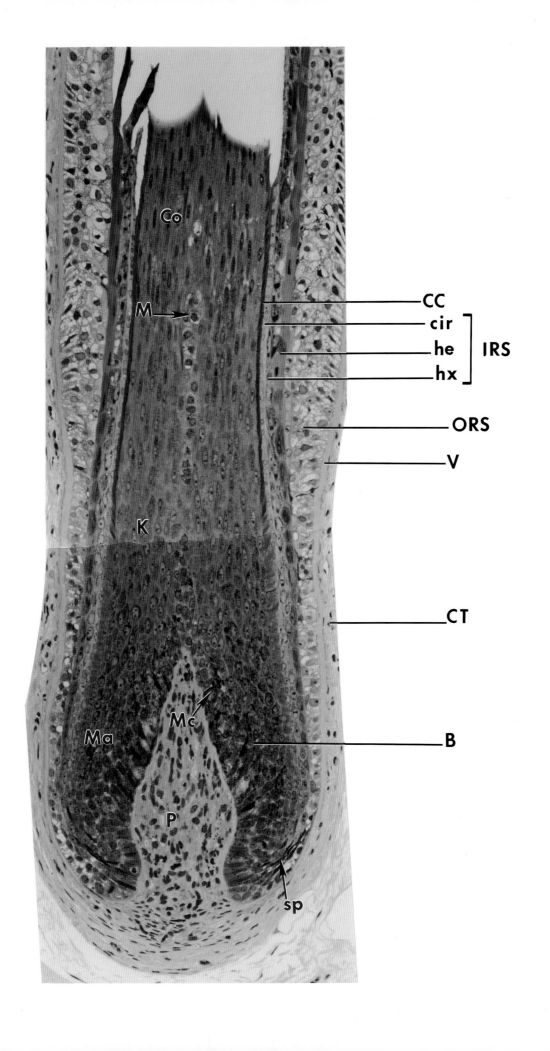

PLATE 155

ANAGEN HAIR FOLLICLE

The bulb is the biochemical laboratory of the follicle. The inner root sheath of each follicle plays a vital role in the formation, or the architecture, of the hair. Henle's layer, on the outside, is the first part to become cornified and is followed by the cuticle of the inner root sheath layer. Together with Huxley's layer, the layers of the inner root sheath form the tips of each hair and help to mold the hair into its final form. The follicle is homologous with a gland that secretes hair material, a holocrine product.

A. Terminal hair follicle from the scalp of a young man. 2-μm plastic section. H and Lee. OM 160x. Figures B, C, and D are enlargements of the areas indicated on this photograph.

B. The cuticle cells of the hair (CH) have become detached from the cuticle of the inner root sheath (CI). Note that the cuticle cells of the hair are larger than those of the inner root sheath. Henle's layer (He), Huxley's layer (Hx), and the cuticle make up the inner root sheath. The vacuolated cells of the outer root sheath (ORS) contain glycogen, lipid, mucopolysaccharide and water. Cortex of the hair (Co). Glassy or vitreous membrane (GM). 2-μm plastic section. H and Lee. OM 630x.

C. At this level of the follicle, above the keratogenous zone (K), the cells that form the cuticle of the hair (CH) are fully cornified in the upper part of the figure and are much larger than those that form the cuticle of the inner root sheath (CI). Henle's layer (He) and Huxley's layer (Hx) are not yet entirely cornified. The outer root sheath (ORS) is very thin here. Note the melanosomes in the cells of the cortex (Co). The melanocytes in the upper part of the bulb provide melanin granules to presumptive cortical and medullary cells, but not to those of the cuticle and the inner root sheath. Near the end of the growth cycle of a follicle, the formation of melanin and of the medulla stops. The last part of the hair is nonmedullated and nonpigmented. 2-μm plastic section. H and Lee. OM 1000x.

D. Matrix cells sweeping upward. Note the melanocytes (M) and the spindle cells (Sp) that separate the cells of the potential inner root sheath (IR) from those of the outer root sheath (ORS). Connective tissue sheath (CT). Glassy membrane (GM). Dermal papilla (P). Basement membrane (BM). 2-μm plastic section. H and Lee. OM 630x.

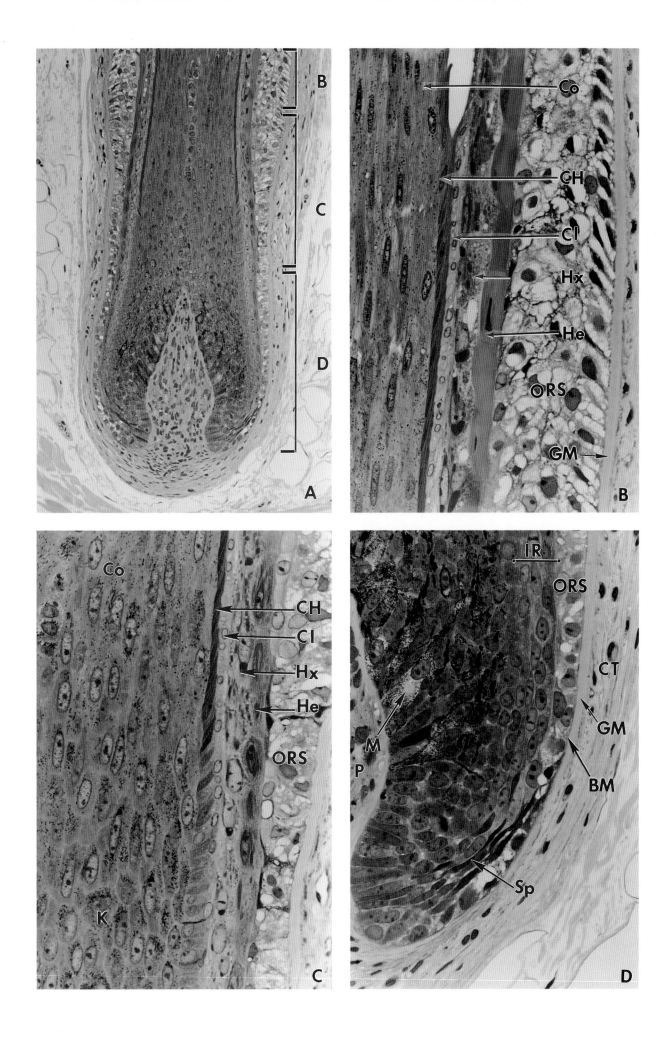

PLATE 156

HAIR FOLLICLE
Black Skin

A. The follicles of kinky hairs are twisted and their bulbs are sharply bent, as shown in this section of a hair follicle from the scalp of a young Black woman. The matrix cells (MC) are stacked in rows as they ascend to the keratogenous zone (K). The outer root sheath (ORS) and the noncellular vitreous membrane (V) are thicker on the inside of the follicular curve. 2-μm plastic section. Giemsa stain. OM 160x.

B. Hair bulb from the scalp of a young Black woman showing excess melanin in the dermal papilla. Melanophages (MP) are full of melanosomes. The clear cells or melanocytes (M) are not very conspicuous. 2-μm plastic section. H and Lee. OM 250x.

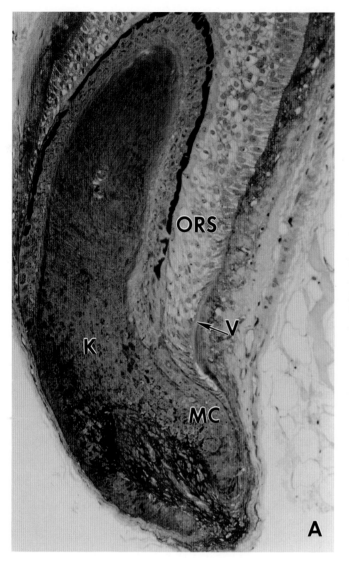

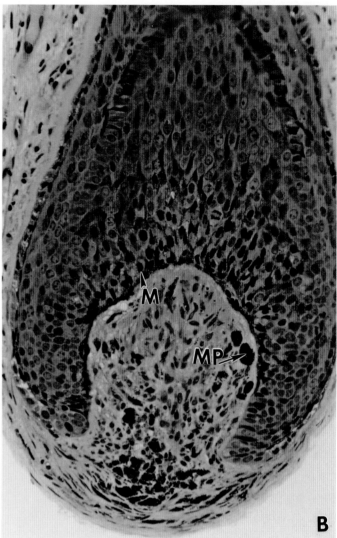

PLATE 157

HAIR FOLLICLE

Black Skin

The terminal hairs of Blacks are crimped or kinky (Figure A), but their intermediate (Figure B) and vellus (Figure C) hairs are straight. The shape of a follicle determines the shape of the hairs it produces.

A. The bulb of a scalp terminal hair follicle of a young Black African woman is abruptly bent. Glassy (vitreous) membrane (GM). Outer root sheath (OR). Henle's layer (He). Huxley's layer (Hx). Cuticle of hair cortex (CH). Matrix (M). Dermal papilla (P). 2-μm plastic section. H and Lee. OM 160x.

B. The bulb of an intermediate hair follicle from the scalp of a young Black African woman produces a straight hair. The follicle contains abundant melanin and its size is between that of a vellus hair (Figure C) and a terminal hair (Figure A). Dermal papilla (P). Henle's layer (He) and Huxley's layer (Hx) of the inner root sheath. Outer root sheath (OR). Glassy membrane (GM). Connective tissue sheath (CT). 2-μm plastic section. H and Lee. OM 160x.

C. Vellus hair follicle from the face of a young Black African woman. The recently formed tip of a vellus hair (arrow), which consists of only the inner root sheath, is faintly colored blue. The inner root sheath, located on both sides of the developing hair, appears to shape or contour the forming hair shaft. A unique characteristic of this vellus hair is that it contains melanin (arrowheads). Dermal papilla (P). 4-μm plastic section. Hale's colloidal iron technique counterstained with nuclear fast red. OM 160x.

D. Early anagen in a follicle of an intermediate hair in the face of a middle-aged White woman shows the hair club (C) surrounded by an epithelial capsule (EC) and the new follicle (NF). Dermal papilla (P). A connective tissue sheath (CT) is just becoming organized. 2-μm plastic section. H and Lee. OM 250x.

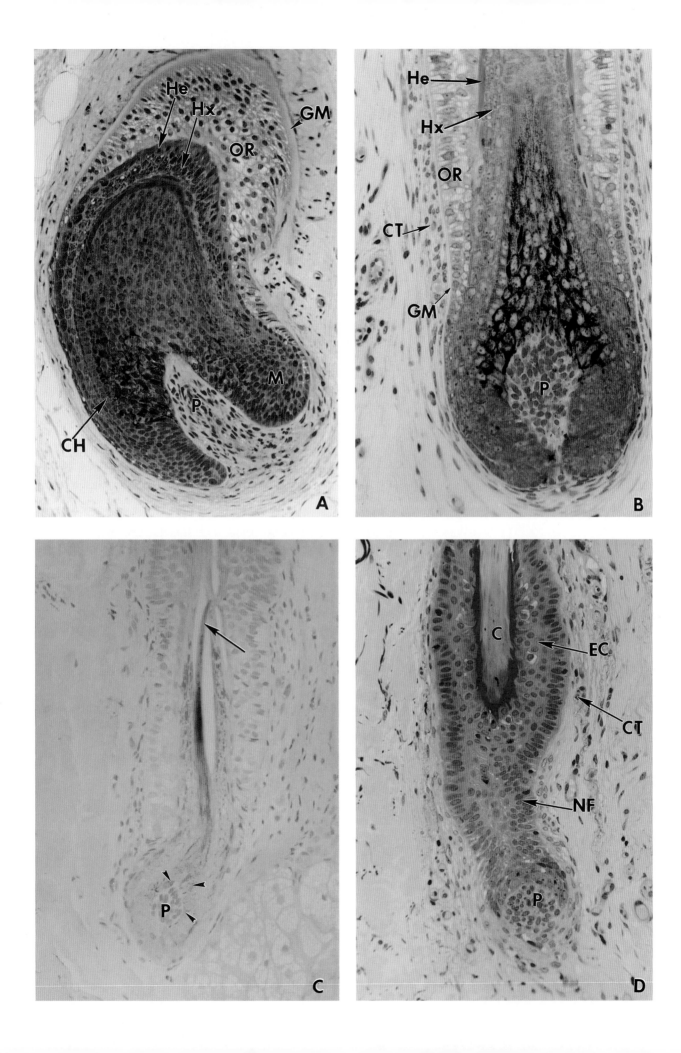

PLATE 158

BEARD HAIR FOLLICLES

At puberty, sex hormones in boys and girls trigger changes in hairs; coarse hairs emerge in the mons pubis and the axilla. The general body hairs and facial hairs are also androgen-dependent. The beard and mustache hairs in men are specific secondary male characteristics.

Beard hair follicles can produce misshapen and sometimes fluted hair. The bulb and the dermal papilla of beard follicles can be slightly or completely divided. If a single follicle contains several hairs, there is a corresponding number of dermal papillae.

A. The bulb of a beard follicle from the chin of a middle-aged Chinese man shows a partial division (arrow) of the dermal papilla (P). The melanocytes have few melanosomes. 2-μm plastic section. H and Lee. OM 160x.

B. The bulbs of curly beard hair follicles are often dumbbell-shaped in section. Papilla (P). From the face of a 48-year-old White man. 2-μm plastic section. H and Lee. OM 160x.

C. Bulb of a beard follicle from the face of a middle-aged Black man. The odd-shaped dermal papilla (P) is partially separated (arrows). Pili multigemini are common in Black men's beards. 2-μm plastic section. H and Lee. OM 160x.

D. Bulb of a beard follicle of a middle-aged White man with a curly, gray beard. Note the protrusions (arrows) in the wall of the dermal papilla (P). The melanocytes have a sparse population of melanosomes. White hair follicles have no melanocytes, and in partially pigmented follicles the melanosomes are incompletely melanized. 2-μm plastic section. H and Lee. OM 160x.

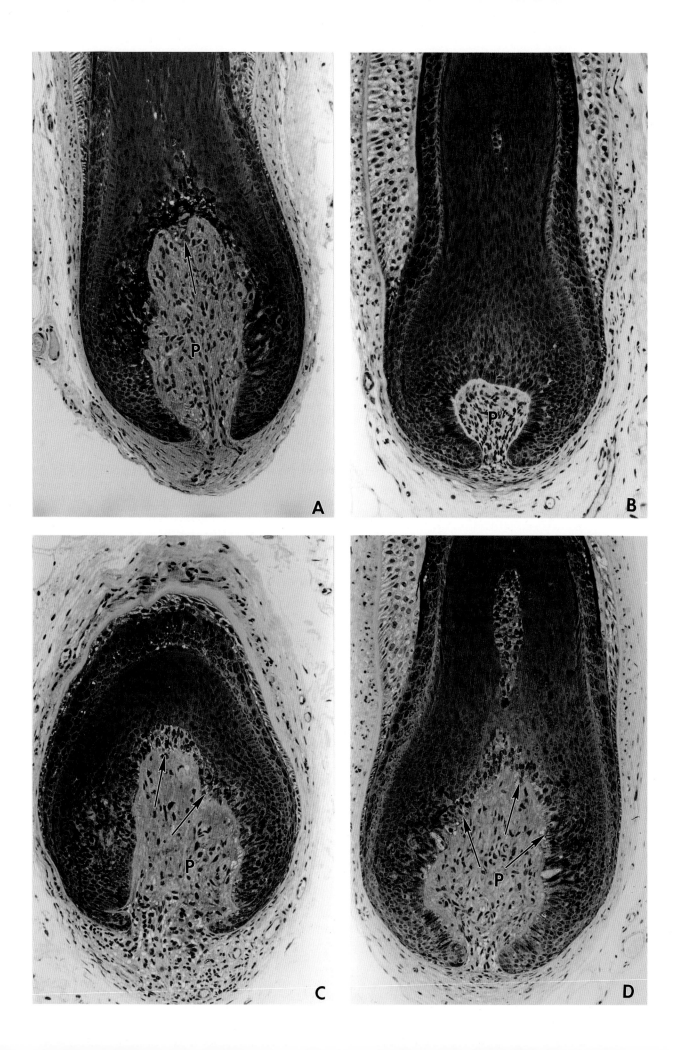

PLATE 159

ANAGEN HAIR FOLLICLE

A. Hair follicle from the scalp of a young White man with extracellular globules of mucopolysaccharide in the dermal papilla (P). In the outer root sheath (OR) the mucopolysaccharide material is intracellular (see Plate 160C). 4-μm plastic section. Hale's colloidal iron technique for mucopolysaccharide. OM 250x.

B. Adjacent section to that in Figure A. The dermal papilla (P) and papilla plate (PP) attain an intense purple color with the Giemsa stain. Note the blood vessels (BV) in the papilla. 2-μm plastic section. Giemsa stain. OM 250x.

C. Hair follicle from the scalp of a young Amerindian woman. The dermal papilla (P) and the basement membrane (BM) are vividly PAS-reactive. The basement membrane separates the papilla from the bulb cells. The presumptive cuticle cells (CC) of the hair and the fibroblasts in the connective tissue sheath (CTS) contain some glycogen granules in their cytoplasm. 2-μm plastic section. PAS. OM 250x.

D. Adjacent section to that in Figure B. The dermal papilla (P) has abundant extracellular material that stains a metachromatic color. The noncellular portion of the dermal papilla, the ground substance, contains small collagenous fibers. 4-μm plastic section. Toluidine blue, pH 5.0. OM 250x.

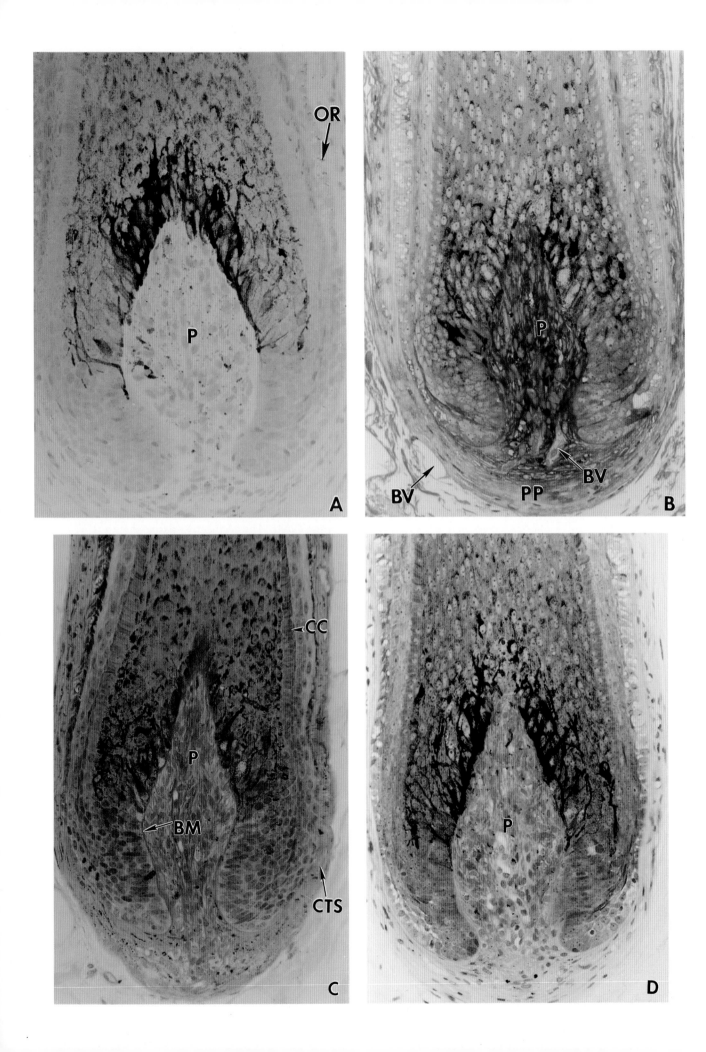

PLATE 160

ANAGEN HAIR FOLLICLE

A. Transverse section in the middle of a terminal hair follicle from the scalp of a young Black woman. The hair has dropped out of the center, leaving behind the cornified inner root sheath (arrow). The outer peripheral cells of the outer root sheath (OR) rest on a thin, PAS-reactive basement membrane (BM). The vitreous membrane (VM) and connective tissue sheath (CTS) are stained a pale color. 4-μm plastic section. PAS counterstained with hematoxylin. OM 160x.

B. Oblique cut through the terminal follicle in the scalp of a young Black African woman. In the center of the figure is the hair surrounded by the cuticle of the cortex (CC), the cuticle of the inner root sheath (CI), Huxley's layer (Hx), and Henle's layer (He). The basal cells of the outer root sheath (BOR) rest on a thin, metachromatic-staining basement membrane (BM) and a thick, unstained vitreous membrane (VM). The connective tissue sheath (CTS) surrounds the vitreous membrane. 2-μm plastic section. Toluidine blue, pH 5.0. OM 250x.

C. Slightly oblique, transverse cut about midway in the length of an anagen hair follicle from the scalp of a young man. There is abundant reactive material inside the cells of the outer root sheath (OR). Henle's layer (He) of the inner root sheath shows a faint reactivity. The trichohyalin granules in Huxley's layer (Hx) are unreactive. Epidermal keratohyalin and the inner root sheath trichohyalin, which appear to be morphologically similar, are biochemically dissimilar. 4-μm plastic section. Hale's colloidal iron technique for mucopolysaccharide counterstained with nuclear fast red. OM 300x.

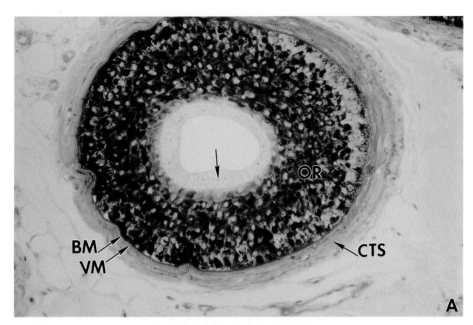

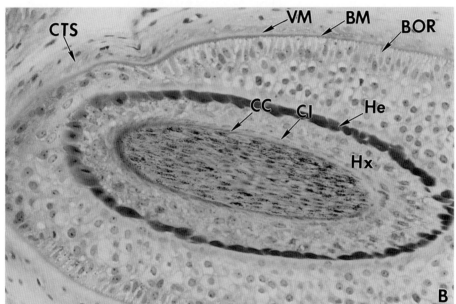

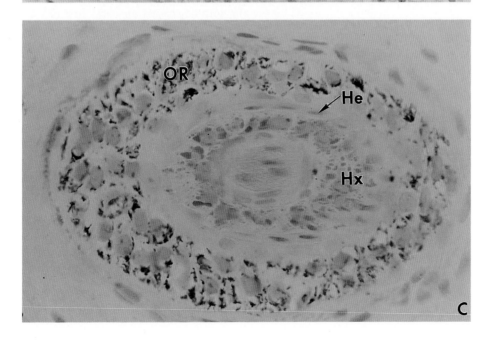

PLATE 161

HAIR SHAFT FUSI

Hausman in 1932 described very small, spindle-shaped spaces in the cortex of the hair shafts, which he called fusi. Before the hair is fully keratinized, these spaces are filled with fluid; as the hair dries out, the fluid is replaced by air. To see fusi well, the hair matrix must be stained a dark color.

A. Transverse section of a terminal hair from the scalp of a young Black African woman. The small, rounded vesicles (F) in the cortex are transversely cut fusi. The medulla (M) is in the center and is composed of large, loose cornified cells. Generally, the medulla is prominent and continuous in the hair of Blacks compared to that of Whites. The cortex is surrounded by a layer of imbricated cortical cuticle scales (Co). Henle's layer (He). Huxley's layer (Hx). Cuticle of the inner root sheath (CI). 2-μm plastic section. Verhoff's elastic fiber technique. OM 160x.

B. In this hair from the scalp of a young man, note the central medulla (M) and the loosened peripheral cortical cuticle cells (Co). The longitudinally cut fusi (F) are oriented parallel to the cortical keratin fibers. Fusi are present in all human hairs, regardless of race. Most hairs float in water due to the presence of air in the medulla and the fusi. 2-μm plastic section. Verhoff's elastic fiber technique. OM 250x.

C. Note the spindle-shaped air sacs, fusi (F), and dense melanosomes in this terminal scalp hair from a young woman. Cortical cuticle (Co). Huxley's layer (Hx) contains green-stained trichohyalin granules. 2-μm plastic section. Fontana-Masson silver technique counterstained with fast green. OM 630x.

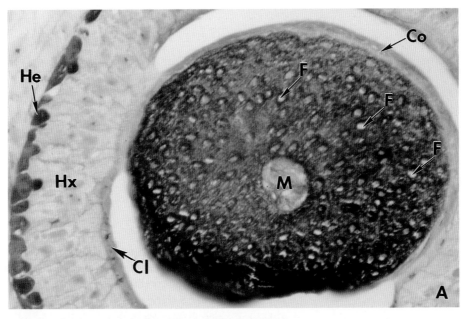

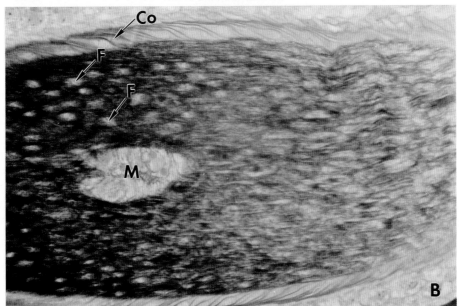

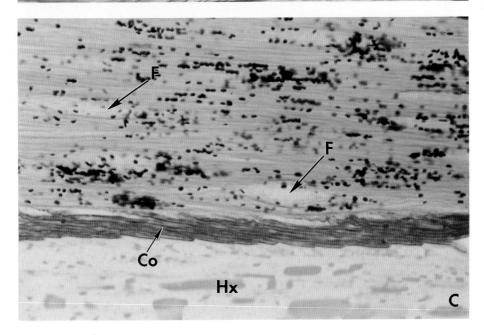

PLATE 162

ANAGEN HAIR FOLLICLE

A. Longitudinal section through a hair follicle just above the keratogenous zone from the scalp of a young White man. Note the imbricated hair cuticle cells (Ct). Melanosomes are confined to the cortex (C). Henle's (He) and Huxley's (Hx) layers of the inner root sheath are also clearly seen. 4-μm plastic section. Fontana-Masson silver technique. OM 630x.

B. In the lower part of the follicle, the cells of the outer root sheath (OR) contain substances that stain a metachromatic color. Basement membrane (BM). Vitreous membrane (V). Connective tissue sheath (Cts). Henle's layer (He). 2-μm plastic section. Toluidine blue, pH 5.0. OM 630x.

C. Outer root sheath of the scalp hair follicle in a young woman. The outer peripheral cells of the outer root sheath rest on a PAS-reactive basement membrane (BM), outside of which is the lightly colored vitreous membrane (VM). On its outside, the vitreous membrane is surrounded by the connective tissue sheath (Cts), in which there are many blood vessels. 4-μm plastic section. PAS counterstained with hematoxylin. OM 1000x.

D. Mitosis is sometimes seen in the basal cells of the outer root sheath, near the upper end of anagen hair follicles. Basement membrane (BM). Vitreous membrane (V). 2-μm plastic section. H and Lee. OM 630x.

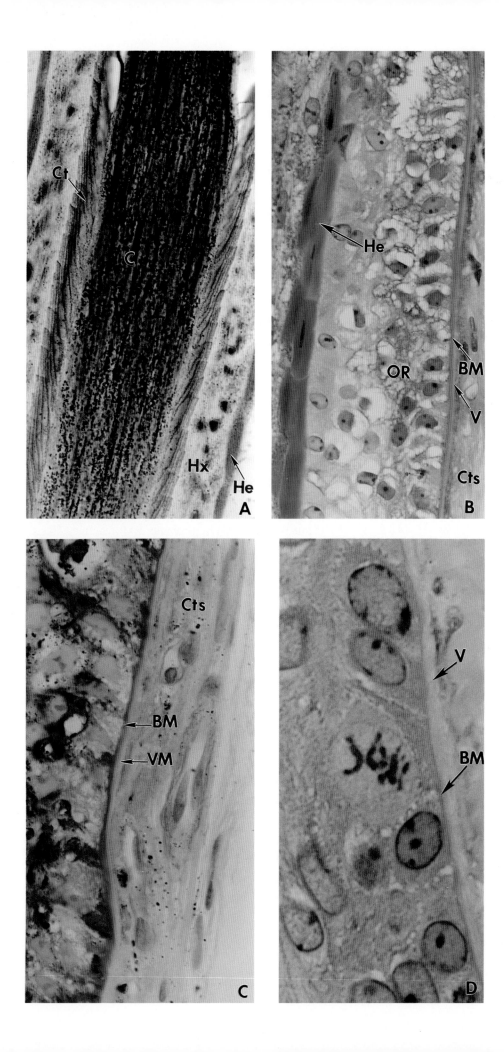

PLATE 163

ANAGEN HAIR FOLLICLE

A. This longitudinal section, midway through an anagen follicle, shows the columnar outer peripheral cells of the outer root sheath (OR). The pleated basement membrane (BM) stains a metachromatic color at this level. Vitreous membrane (VM). 2-μm plastic section. Toluidine blue, pH 5.0. OM 630x.

B. Basal cells of the outer root sheath (OR) of the same follicle as in Figure A. Glycogen stains bright red. The basal cells rest on a PAS-reactive basement membrane (BM). Vitreous membrane (VM). 4-μm plastic section. PAS counterstained with hematoxylin. OM 1000x.

C. Oblique cut midway through a follicle from the scalp of a middle-aged White man. The circular pleats of the basement membrane (BM) are conspicuously PAS-reactive, but the thick vitreous membrane (VM) is minimally PAS-reactive. This skin specimen was stored in 10% formalin for 2 years before it was embedded in glycolmethacrylate, perhaps accounting for the artifacts. 4-μm plastic section. PAS counterstained with hematoxylin. OM 630x.

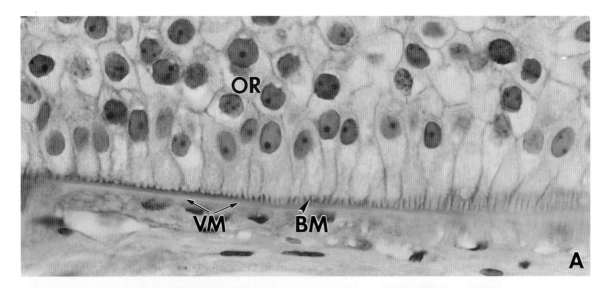

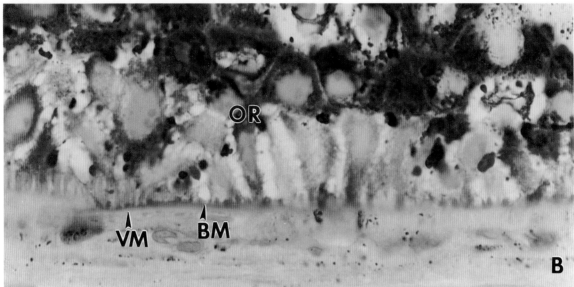

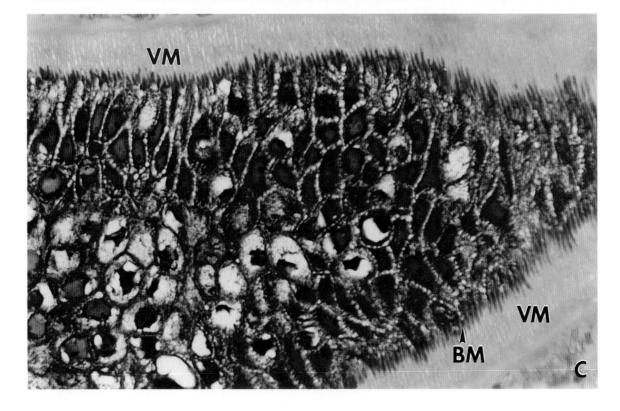

PLATE 164

INNER ROOT SHEATH

A. This section of the scalp of a young woman shows that the cornified inner root sheath is discharged inside the pilosebaceous canal. The horny cells of Henle's layer (He) stain darker than those of Huxley's layer (Hx). Epidermis (Ep). 2-μm plastic section. H and Lee. OM 250x.

B. In the same section as in Figure A, note what happens to the inner root sheath just below the entrance of the sebaceous glands (S). Henle's layer (He) gives rise to the dark-red-stained corrugations (C); Huxley's layer (Hx) forms the flimsy surface layer over the corrugations. The cuticle of the inner root sheath (CIR) disappears. 2-μm plastic section. H and Lee. OM 250x.

C. In this longitudinally cut hair follicle from the scalp of a 20-year-old man, the entire inner root sheath (IR) is stained black (positive for alkaline phosphatase); its upper end extends to the infundibulum just below the entrance of the sebaceous glands (S). Blood vessels are stained black. 30-μm frozen section. Gomori's alkaline phosphatase technique. OM 160x.

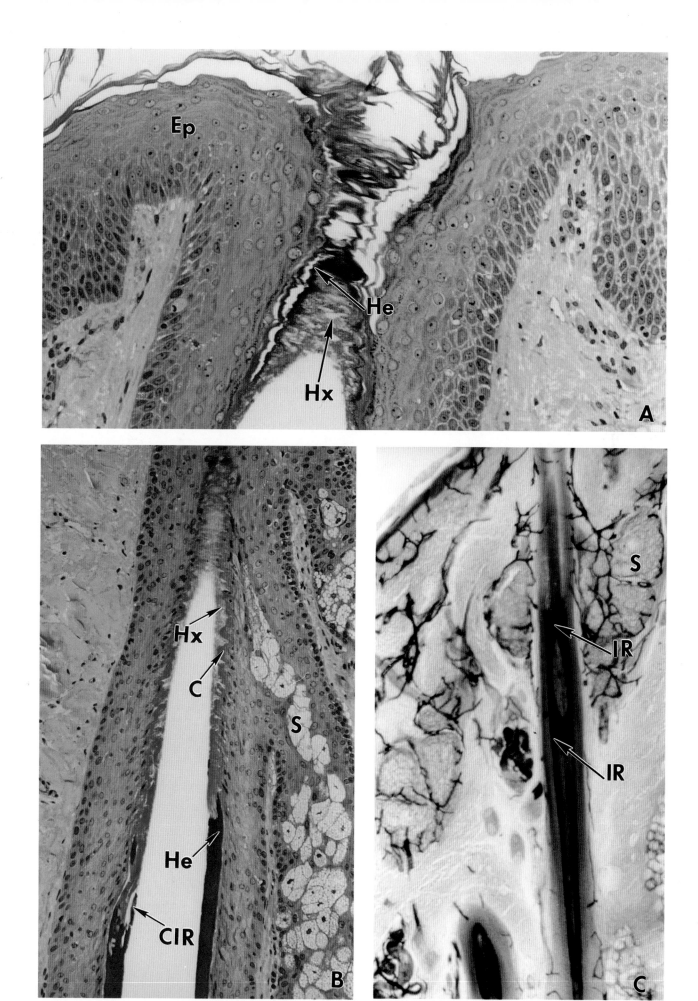

PLATE 165

INNER ROOT SHEATH

The inner root sheath cornifies and is ultimately lost inside the infundibulum of the follicle as the hair emerges. This montage of a scalp hair follicle from a young woman shows the parts of the inner root sheath just below the entrance of the sebaceous gland (S). Corrugations are formed by Henle's layer (He). Huxley's layer (Hx) forms the diaphanous part of the corrugations. There is no trace of the cuticle of the inner root sheath. 2-μm plastic section. H and Lee. OM 250x.

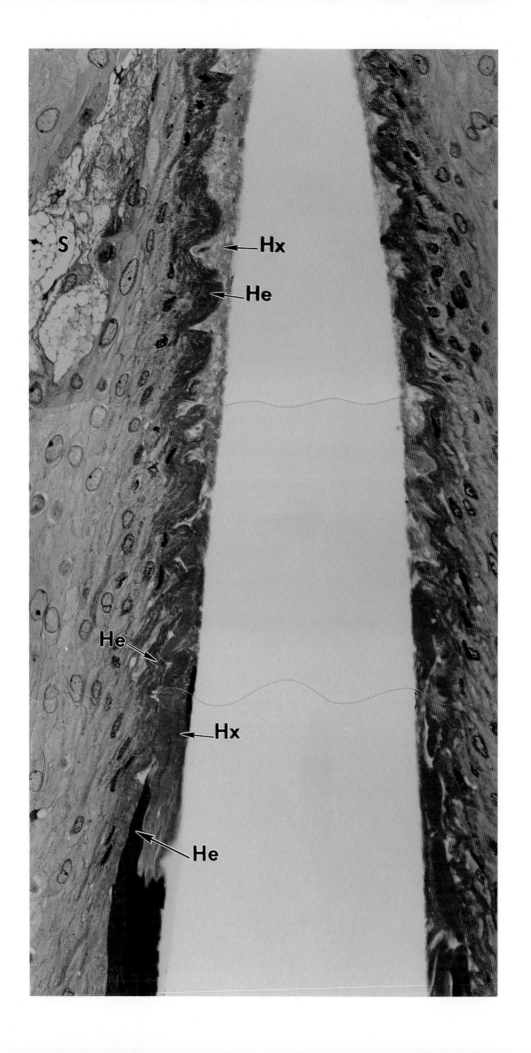

PLATE 166

HAIR GROWTH CYCLE
Three Stages

Hair follicles have periods of growth and quiescence, known collectively as hair growth cycles. An understanding of hair growth cycles is the key to an understanding of the biology of hair growth.

Anagen. The follicle is divided into an upper and a lower part; the permanent upper portion is located above the bulge and the transient lower part is below the bulge. The bulge is a bump on the upper part of the follicle's outer root sheath, just below the entrance of the sebaceous glands. After the hair follicle has grown for a period of time, it discards the transient portion and enters into catagen, which is followed by telogen, a period of rest or quiescence. Adjacent follicles may have different periods of growth and quiescence (hair growth cycles). These cycles are established in utero.

Catagen. When the follicle is nearing the end of its growth period and prepares to enter catagen, the matrix cells stop differentiating and become a column of cells. Melanocytes stop functioning so that the last segment of each hair formed is white. The club is then formed in the keratogenous zone and mitosis stops in the matrix cells. The transient part of the follicle below the bulge degenerates, and the dermal papilla follows the retreat of the follicle, which shrinks to one-third of its original size. In the meantime, the inner root sheath metamorphoses into an anchoring substance that secures the hair club into the epithelial capsule. The follicle is surrounded by a row of macrophages that clean up the debris from the follicle.

Telogen. The quiescent follicle represents what remains of the original follicle (the permanent part) after catagen. During telogen, the follicles remain quiescent for variable periods of time. The length of telogen varies from area to area and gets longer with aging.

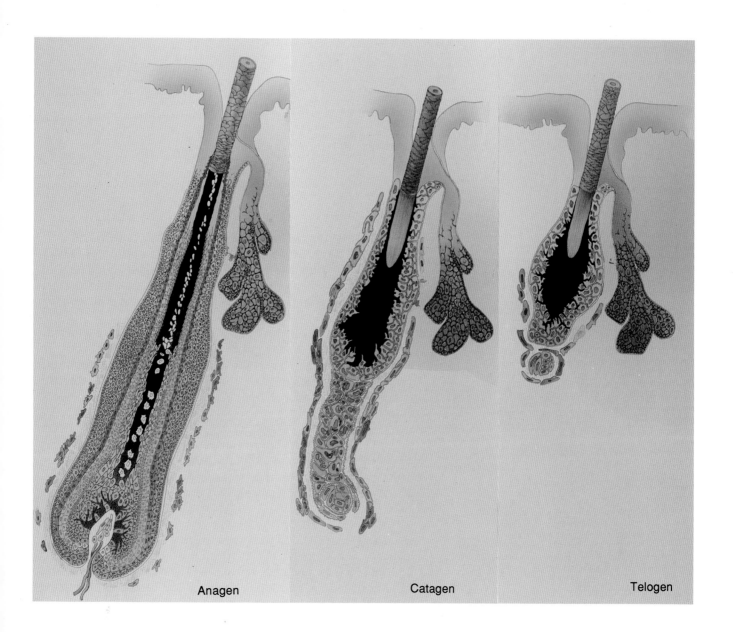

Anagen   Catagen   Telogen

PLATE 167

HAIR FOLLICLES

All of the events in the formation of the first hair follicles and their conversion from active to resting follicles are templates for follicular activity in postnatal life. The follicles cycle throughout life with alternating periods of growth and quiescence. Each follicle has its own growth cycle that is independent of that of other follicles.

A. Two lanugo follicles in the labia minora of an 8-month fetal girl. The labia minora, usually glabrous in women, have lanugo hairs during fetal life; these gradually disappear before and after birth. There are acetylcholinesterase-containing nerves around the two follicles. 20-μm frozen section. Koelle's acetylcholinesterase technique. OM 120x.

B and C. Hair follicles in early anagen growing from telogen follicles in the scalp of a 6-month fetus. Hair growth cycles begin during fetal life; there are three or more hair growth cycles before birth. 20-μm frozen section. Roman's AOV elastic fiber technique. OM 100x.

D. In this frozen section from the scalp of a young man, a terminal hair follicle in anagen (A) is on the left of the one in telogen (T). The short follicle and club hair on the right are the characteristic features of resting, or telogen, follicles. The dermal papilla (P) is below the epithelial capsule, around the club of the follicle, in telogen. The sebaceous (S) and eccrine (E) sweat glands are surrounded by black-stained blood vessels. Arrectores pilorum muscles (AP) are very large. 20-μm frozen section. Gomori's alkaline phosphatase technique. OM 120x.

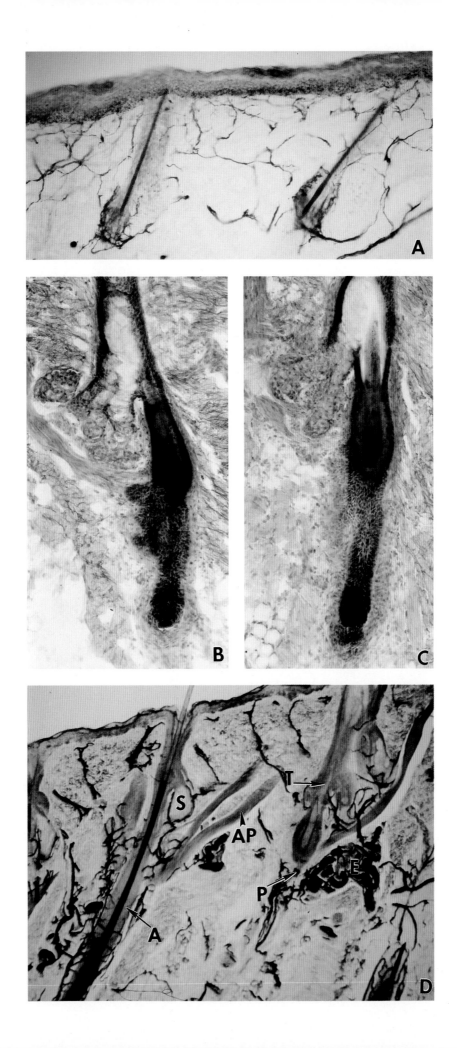

PLATE 168

HAIR FOLLICLES

A. Quiescent (telogen) hair follicle from the scalp of a young White man. Quiescent periods range from very short in the scalp to long in some parts of the body. Note the club hair (CH) and the surrounding epithelial capsule (EC). The remains of the connective tissue sheath (arrows) form a trail below the dermal papilla (P). Basement membrane (BM). 2-μm plastic section. H and Lee. OM 160x.

B. The club hair (CH) is surrounded and anchored by the remains of the inner root sheath (IRS). There is a conspicuous difference in the tinctorial properties of the hair club and the inner root sheath. The cells of the epithelial capsule (EC) make contact in a zipper-like fashion (arrow). 2-μm plastic section. H and Lee. OM 1250x.

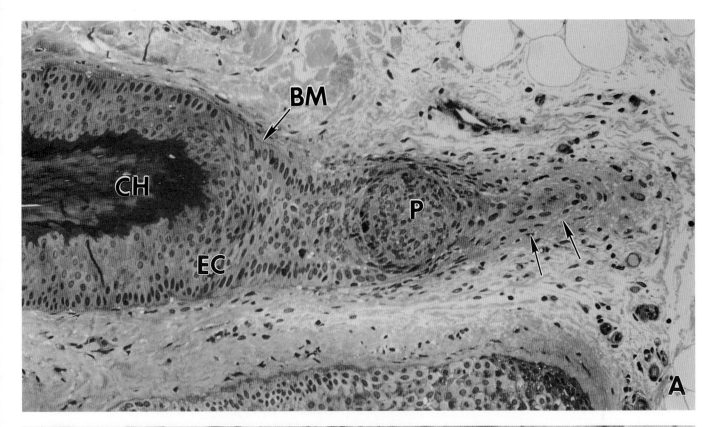

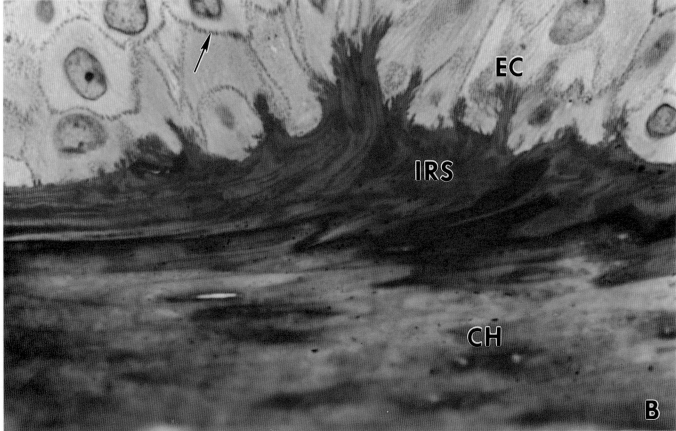

PLATE 169

HAIR FOLLICLES

A. Upper right quadrant of the dermal papilla (P) of an anagen follicle from the scalp of a young man. The thick basement membrane (BM) appears to be continuous with the material between the papilla cells. The cytoplasm of the papilla cells remains unstained. Large melanocytes (M) are crowded above the upper half or two-thirds of the dermal papilla. Follicles that produce large hairs have large bulbs and dermal papillae, and vice versa. 4-μm plastic section. PAS counterstained with hematoxylin. OM 1260x.

B. Follicular growth comes to a halt in catagen, and the follicle undergoes striking structural and functional changes. The melanocytes contract their dendrites and melanogenesis stops. In this catagen follicle, melanin is being spilled and taken up by the macrophages (MP) in the connective tissue trail below the dermal papilla (P). The cellular remains of the follicle are still surrounded by a PAS-reactive basement membrane (BM). The dermal papilla is in contact with the receding follicle; it still contains blood vessels (BV) and its crowded cells are smaller than the papilla cells in anagen follicles. 4-μm plastic section. PAS counterstained with hematoxylin. OM 630x.

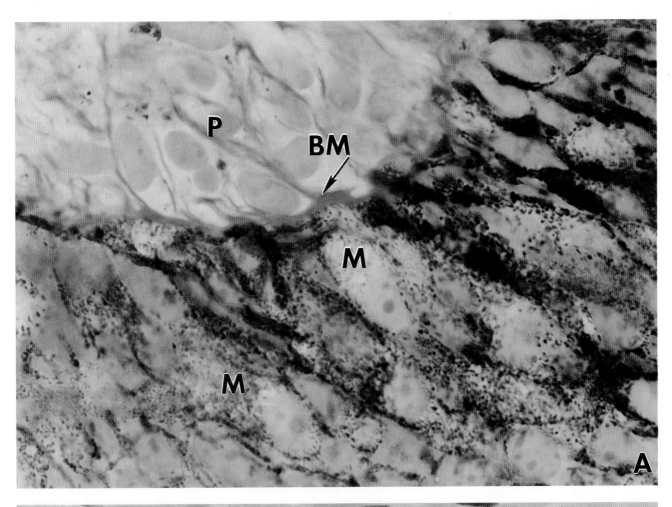

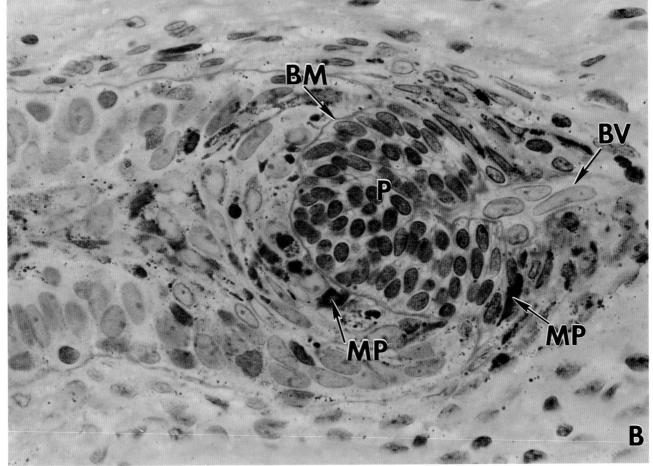

PLATE 170

HAIR FOLLICLES

A. The dermal papilla (P) of a scalp hair follicle in catagen is a distance away from the receding hair follicle; a thin column of degenerating cells (arrows) retains contact between the dermal papilla and the follicle (F). The vitreous membrane (V) zigzags around what remains of the follicle's bulb. There are many blood vessels (B) in the connective tissue sheath (CT). 10-μm paraffin section. Gomori's acid phosphatase technique. OM 120x.

B. Scalp hair follicle in late catagen. The dermal papilla (P) has risen up to the retreating lower (transient) part of the follicle (F). A crinkly vitreous membrane (V) surrounds the follicle. Club hair (CH). Connective tissue sheath (CT). 10-μm paraffin section. H and E. OM 160x.

C. A dermal papilla (P) is clearly evident in a vellus follicle in early anagen. The tip of this hair (arrow) has just been formed; it is composed entirely of inner root sheath. The club hair (CH) of the previous follicle is still inside the permanent part of the follicle. Only two small anlagen (A) of sebaceous glands are present. The most conspicuous elements of the new follicle are the cornifying cells of Henle's layer (He) of the inner root sheath. The upper part of the dermis in this skin from the face of a young man shows pronounced photodamage. 4-μm plastic section. Verhoff's elastic fiber technique. OM 120x.

D. The nerves of this arrector pili muscle (AP) branch from the nerves around the follicle (F), and all the nerves are reactive for acetylcholinesterase. 30-μm frozen section. Koelle's acetylcholinesterase technique. OM 250x.

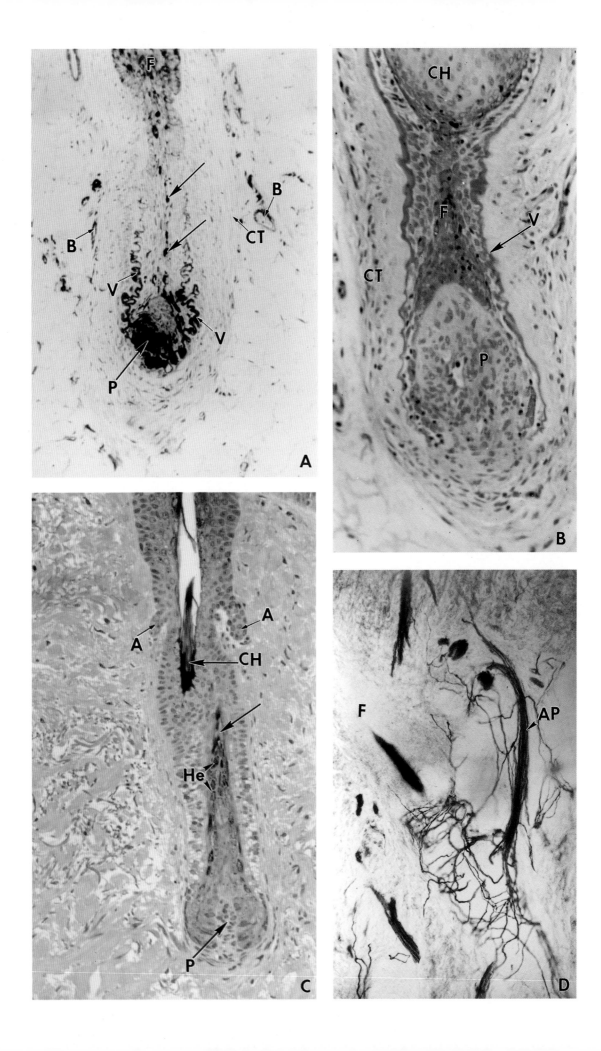

PLATE 171

ARRECTOR PILI MUSCLE

All hair follicles have a strap of smooth muscle attached to the bulge, a bump on the upper part of the follicle's outer root sheath below the sebaceous glands. It has recently been shown that the bulge of the telogen hair follicle contains the stem cells for the future anagen follicle. This means that the cells that form the hair germ of early anagen follicles migrate from the bulge to the epithelial capsule. Thus, the bulge has attained a significance that overshadows its minor anatomical role as the area for the attachment of the arrectores pilorum muscles.

A. Transverse section through an arrector pili muscle. Some of the muscle cells characteristically stain a lighter color than others. Arrectores pilorum muscles are large and long in human skin. 2-μm plastic section. H and Lee. OM 630x.

B. Oblique section through an arrector pili muscle from the scalp of a young woman. Long smooth muscle cells with centrally located nuclei have some fat cells (arrow) between them. It is normal to have fat between the smooth muscle cells. 2-μm plastic section. H and Lee. OM 630x.

C. Transverse section through the smooth muscle cells of an arrector pili muscle from the sun-damaged face of a 73-year-old man. Some of the muscle cells have vacuoles (V) under the sarcolemma. This appears to be due to fatty degeneration of muscle cells. 2-μm plastic section. H and Lee. OM 1000x.

D. Transverse section through an arrector pili muscle from the scalp of a young woman. The sarcolemma of the smooth muscle cells is PAS-reactive, and some muscle cells have glycogen granules in the sarcoplasm. 4-μm plastic section. PAS counterstained with hematoxylin. OM 250x.

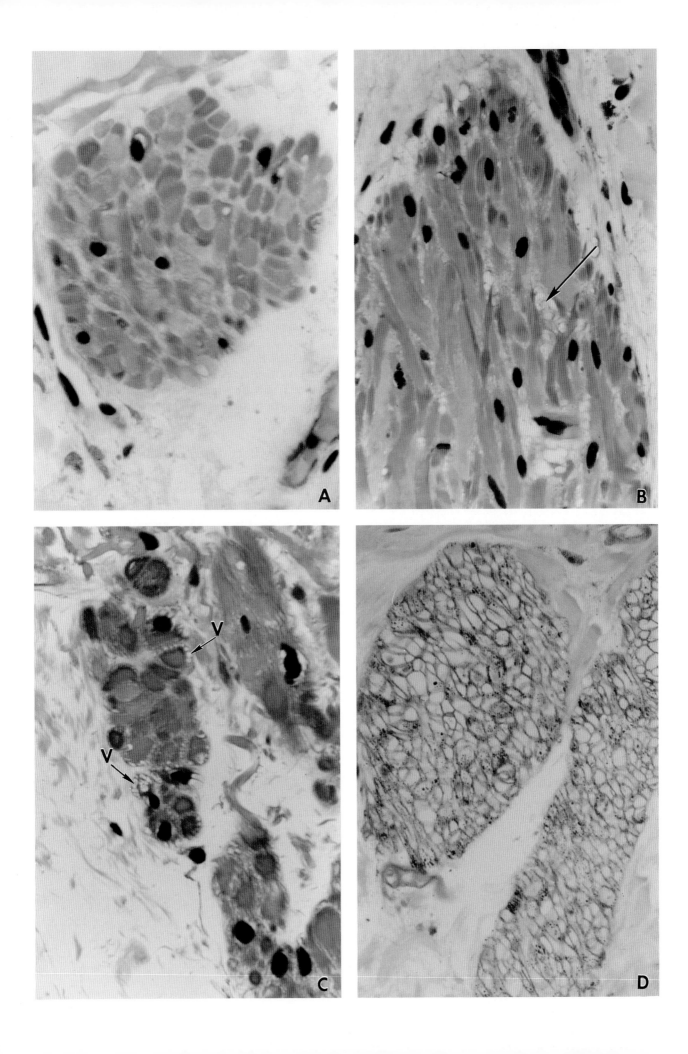

PLATE 172

ARRECTOR PILI MUSCLE

A. Oblique section through an arrector pili muscle with many glycogen globules in the sarcoplasm. 4-μm plastic section. PAS counterstained with hematoxylin. OM 630x.

B. Reticulin fibers are numerous around all smooth muscle cells. Thick, coarse fibers are oriented longitudinally along the axis of the cells, and very fine fibers are wrapped loosely around each muscle cell. 4-μm plastic section. Gridley's reticulin fiber technique. OM 1000x.

C. Arrector pili muscle from the scalp of a young White man is strongly reactive for acetylcholinesterase and is supplied by acetylcholinesterase-reactive nerves (arrows). 15-μm frozen section. Koelle's acetylcholinesterase technique. OM 250x.

D. Skeletal muscle fibers are present, notably in the skin of the head and the scrotum. This muscle fiber, with the characteristic cross banding, is from the face of a 57-year-old White man. 2-μm plastic section. H and Lee. OM 630x.

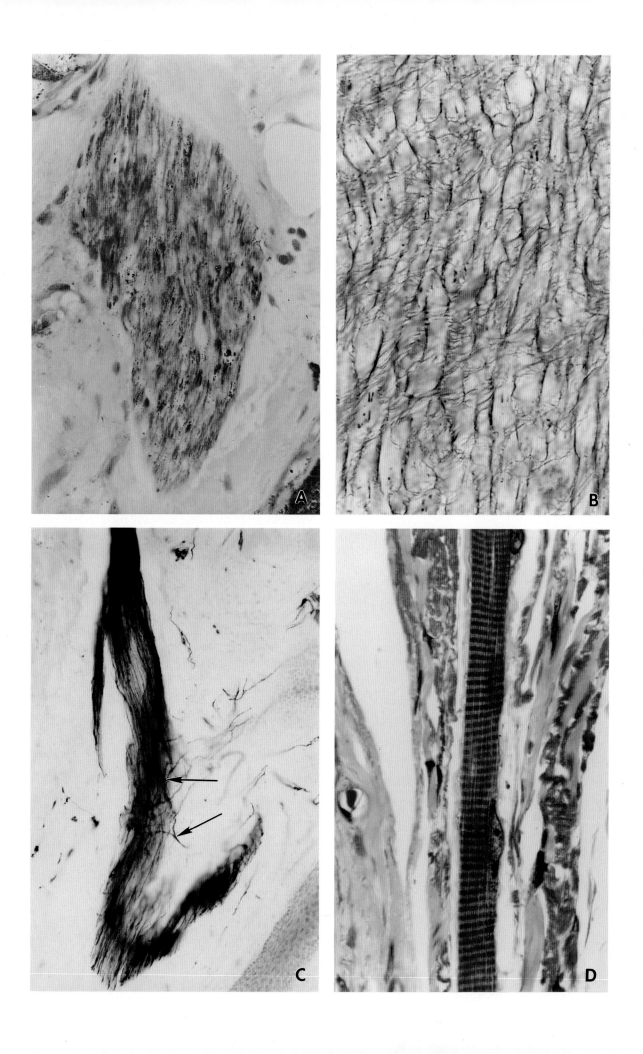

PLATE 173

HAIR
Elastic Fibers

A. The upper part (permanent portion) of the hair follicles is anchored to the dermis by elastic fibers; the lower part, in the papillae adiposae of the hypodermis, has few or no elastic fibers. This frozen section from the scalp of a young White man is cut parasagittally. Sebaceous glands (arrow) may also be anchored in the dermis by delicate elastic fibers. 40-μm frozen section. Roman's AOV elastic fiber technique. OM 250x.

B. In thin sections, only small fragments of elastic fibers can be seen around the upper permanent portion of the hair follicles. 4-μm plastic section. Weigert's elastic fiber technique. OM 400x.

C. Frontal section of the scalp of a young White man, showing the disposition and abundance of elastic fibers around the groups of hair follicles. The scalp and face contain the greatest amount of elastic fibers. 40-μm frozen section. Roman's AOV elastic fiber technique. OM 160x.

D. Arao-Perkins body (arrow) at the base of the dermal papilla of a terminal hair follicle in the scalp of a 13-year-old boy. Not much is known about Arao-Perkins bodies except that they can be demonstrated best in the scalp follicles of preadolescent and adolescent people. 20-μm frozen section. Roman's AOV elastic fiber technique. Courtesy of Prof. T. Arao.

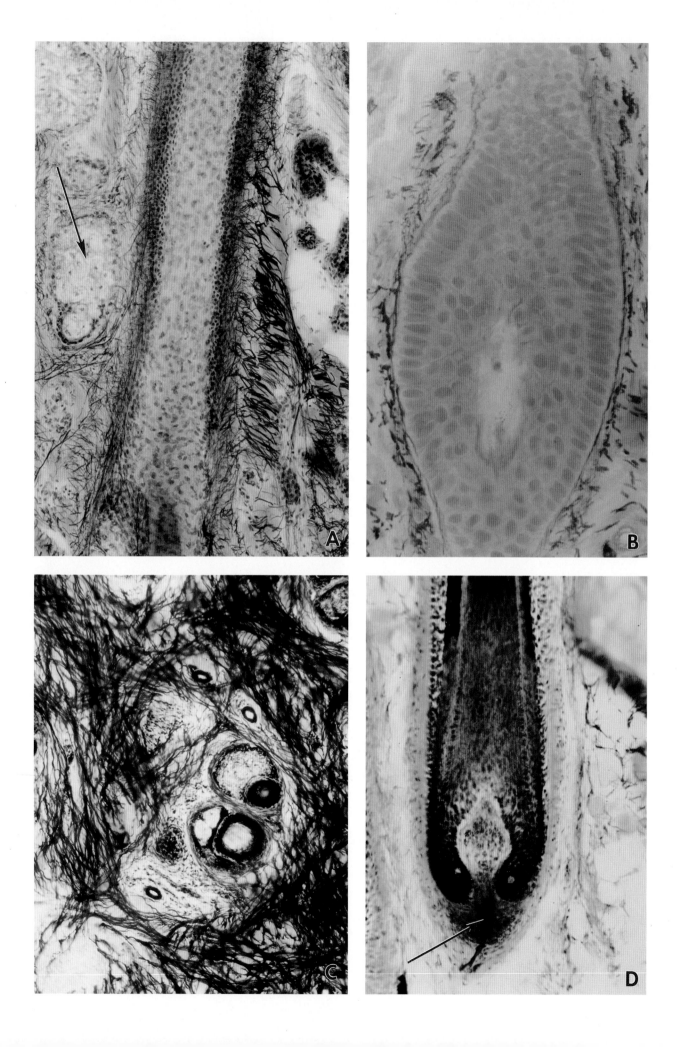

PLATE 174

HAIR FOLLICLES
Blood Vessels

The endothelium of the capillaries and arterioles is easily visualized by using the alkaline phosphatase technique. Thick frozen sections clearly show the rich vascular plexus around hair follicles. Vascularization is particularly abundant in the upper and lower parts of the follicle

A. Hair follicles in the scalp of a 21-year-old man. The blood vessels (stained black) are numerous around the lower parts of the follicles, which rest in the papillae adiposae of the hypodermis (Hy), and the uppermost regions, including the sebaceous glands (S). 20-μm frozen section. Gomori's alkaline phosphatase technique. OM 40x.

B. Basal portion of hair follicles in the fatty layer of the scalp of a 20-year-old man. Blood vessels penetrate the dermal papilla (arrow) of one of the follicles. 20-μm frozen section. Gomori's alkaline phosphatase technique. OM 40x.

C. Blood vessels inside the dermal papilla (P) in the bulb of a terminal hair follicle in the scalp of a 20-year-old man. A bouquet of blood vessels springs from where the Arao-Perkins body is usually located (arrow). 40-μm frozen section. Gomori's alkaline phosphatase technique counterstained with H and E. OM 100x.

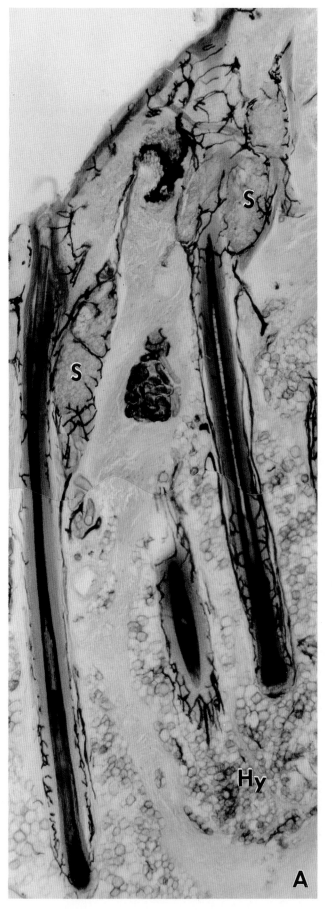

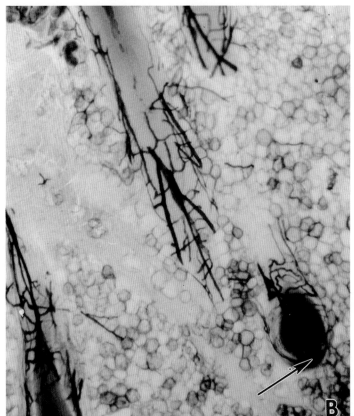

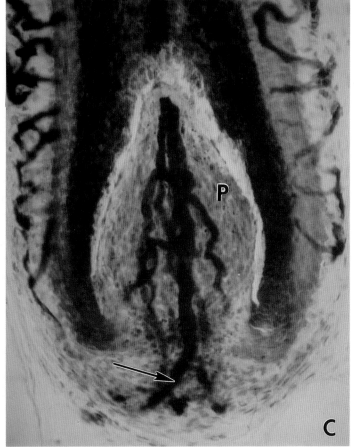

PLATE 175

BALDNESS

The construction of hairs by their follicles is so complicated that it is not surprising that sometimes things go astray in spite of the efficacy of the established programming. Follicles sometimes form abnormal hairs. Although the scalp hair follicles grow well in spite of hormonal milieu (they grow well in women, men, and eunuchs) and do not seem to be androgen-dependent, the scalp of some men, who have a genetic predisposition for baldness and the proper amounts of androgens, becomes bald. Thus, baldness is a secondary male sex characteristic that is dependent on androgen and/or its metabolites. Women can also become bald.

A. This is thought to be a hair follicle in anagen that contains the remains of the club and inner root sheath (arrow) of the previous telogen follicle. Such fortuitous oddities do not occur often. From the face of a 24-year-old White man. 4-μm plastic section. Verhoff's elastic fiber technique. OM 500x.

B. This hair follicle from the bald scalp of a middle-aged man is structurally abnormal. The most conspicuous abnormalities are the disarray of Henle's layer (He) and the disorder in the matrix cells (M). Dermal papilla (P). Outer root sheath (OR). 2-μm plastic section. H and Lee. OM 250x.

C. The arrectores pilorum muscles in bald scalps have an altered tinctorial nature. The increased amount of fat between the muscle fibers (arrows) may indicate fatty infiltration. 2-μm plastic section. H and Lee. OM 630x.

D. The smooth muscle cells (arrows) of the arrectores pilorum muscles in bald scalps sometimes tend to scatter in the connective tissue. 2-μm plastic section. H and Lee. OM 630x.

E. Very large multinucleated giant cells, often aggregated, may occur in bald scalps. These multinucleated giant cells are grossly vacuolated at their periphery, and the one in the center contains the remains of a hair (arrow). Hair fragments in the dermis are nearly always accompanied by multinucleated giant cells. 2-μm plastic section. H and Lee. OM 800x.

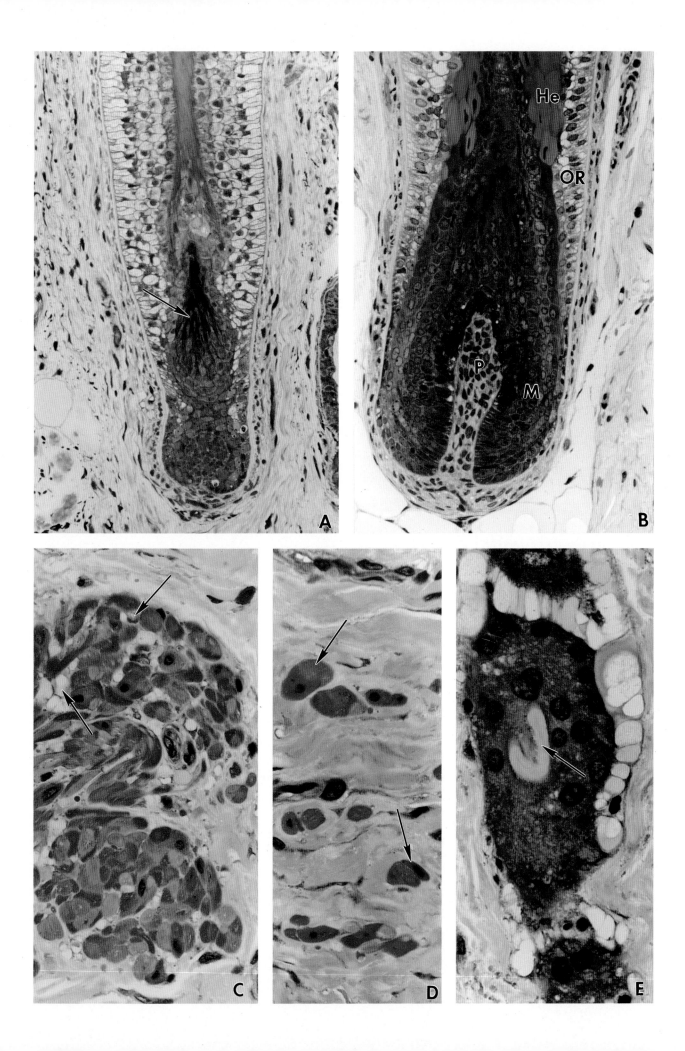

Hypodermis

Man is a fatty animal. The surface of the skin is oily, and with the exception of the eyelids and the male genitalia, a layer of fat occurs over most of the body. The primary functions of the fatty layer are thermoregulation, cushioning against mechanical trauma, contouring the body, filling space, and, most importantly, serving as a readily available source of energy. The fatty layer (hypodermis) differs in thickness with sex, race, and individual nutritional and hormonal status.

PLATE 176

HYPODERMIS

Male and Female

Scarcely anyone today has studied the hypodermal fatty layer, except for the German investigators Nürnberger and Müller. The hypodermis consists of three fatty layers (1,2,3) separated by connective tissue sheaths (retinacula cutis). The top layer, which is thicker in women than in men, has fewer connective tissue septa in women than in men, and the chambers that the retinacula separate are larger in women than in men. These differences are androgen-dependent; in the skin of fetuses younger than 7 to 8 months there are no male and female differences, and the top layer of the hypodermis favors the architecture found in female fetuses. The sex differences appear at the end of the third trimester. In feminized men, the architecture of the top hypodermal layer is like that of women. The papillae adiposae, similar in men and women, are extensions of the upper fatty layer. The bulbs of the larger hair follicles, the glomeruli of the sweat glands, blood vessels, and nerves rest in these superficial fatty chambers.

These diagrams and photographs show the differences that exist in the top fatty layer between men and women.

A. Diagram of the hypodermal layers (1,2,3) showing the female pattern. Note the large, standing fat-cell chambers (F) separated by retinacula (R). Papillae adiposae (P). Redrawn from a diagram courtesy of Prof. F. Nürnberger.

B. This section, from the thigh, shows the typical female pattern of the top hypodermal layer with large, standing fat-cell chambers (F) and radially disposed septa of connective tissue. Retinacula (R). 100-μm paraffin section unstained and viewed under polarized light. Courtesy of Prof. F. Nürnberger.

C. Diagram of the hypodermal layers (1,2,3) showing the male pattern. The pattern shows rather small, polygonal fat-cell chambers (F) with crisscrossing connective tissue septa, or retinacula (R). The superficial extensions of the fatty chambers end in papillae adiposae (P). The papillae adiposae become larger in the elderly. Redrawn from a diagram courtesy of Prof. F. Nürnberger.

D. This section, from the thigh of a 45-year-old man, shows the typical male pattern in the hypodermis. Polarized light shows the birefringent retinacula cutis (R) around the small, polygonal fat chambers (F). 100-μm paraffin section. Courtesy of Prof. F. Nürnberger.

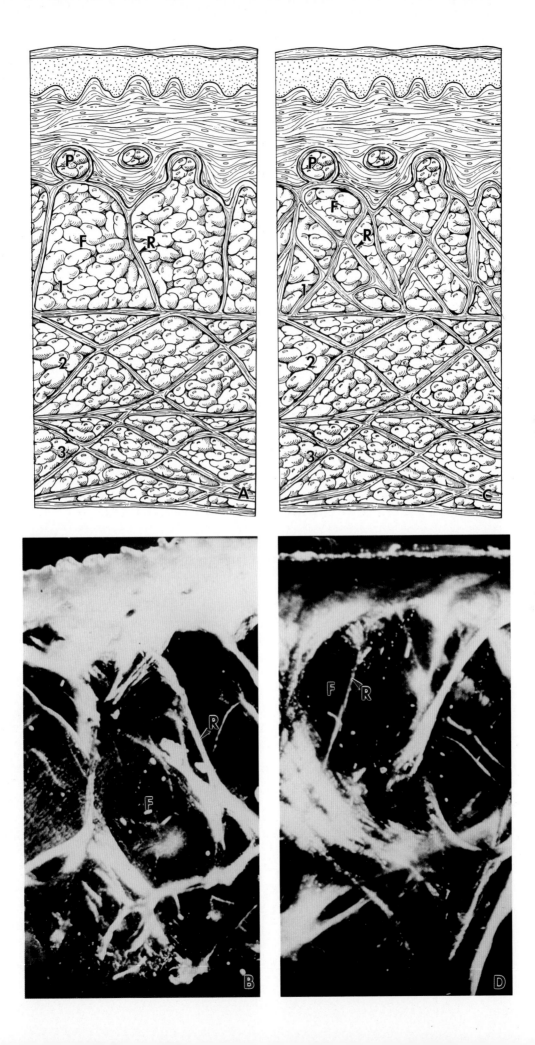

PLATE 177

ADIPOCYTES

A. Fatty tissue in the facial skin of a young man. Blood vessels (arrows) are numerous between the fat-laden, balloon-like adipocytes (A). 2-μm plastic section. Regaud's iron hematoxylin. OM 160x.

B. Adipocyte with characteristic bubble-like inclusions (arrow) in or near the nucleus (N). Although this is not known with certainty, the "nuclear" bubbles may be fatty globules in the cytoplasm that push against the nuclear membrane. 4-μm plastic section. Weigert's elastic fiber technique. OM 250x.

C. This typical adipocyte forms a signet ring-like structure. The cell has a thin plasma membrane and normal dark-staining granules (arrow) in the cytoplasm. Nucleus (N). 4-μm plastic section. Weigert's elastic fiber technique. OM 250x.

D. Nucleus of an undifferentiated adipocyte between mature fat cells with a large bubble-like sphere (arrow). Nucleus (N). 4-μm plastic section. Weigert's elastic fiber technique. OM 400x.

E. Immature adipocyte with several bubble-like spheres (arrow); the bubble inclusions are rarely seen in cells other than those of skin hypodermis. 4-μm plastic section. Weigert's elastic fiber technique. OM 400x.

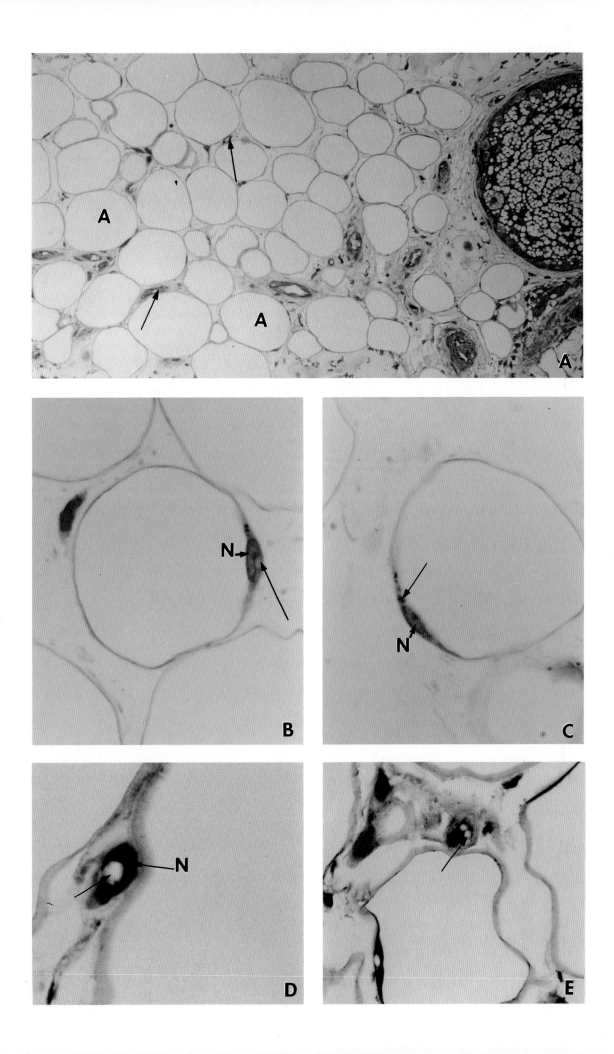

PLATE 178

ADIPOCYTES

A. When the plasma membrane of an adipocyte is spongy (arrows), the cell is in transition; the adipocyte could be an immature cell, or a mature cell in the process of losing or accumulating its fat. The adipocyte nucleus appears to have a large, empty bubble (B). 2-μm plastic section. Regaud's iron hematoxylin. OM 630x.

B. This adipocyte is also in transition with a spongy plasma membrane (arrows). It is either becoming differentiated or losing its fat content. Sometimes the fat contains flocculent or particulate material (P). 2-μm plastic section. Regaud's iron hematoxylin. OM 630x.

C. Plasma membrane of an adipocyte with flocculent material attached to its outer border (arrows). 4-μm plastic section. Azure–eosin stain. OM 400x.

D. There are blood vessels (B) and mast cells (M) in the interstices between mature adipocytes. 2-μm plastic section. Azure–eosin stain. OM 400x.

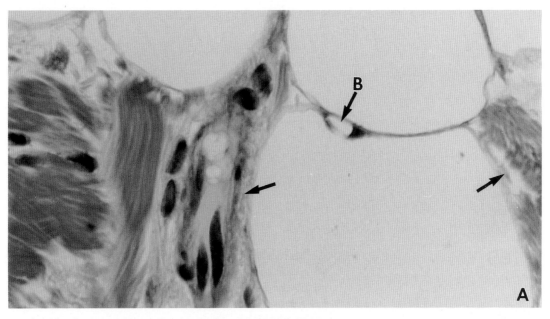

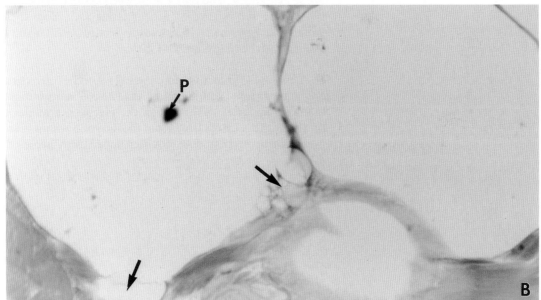

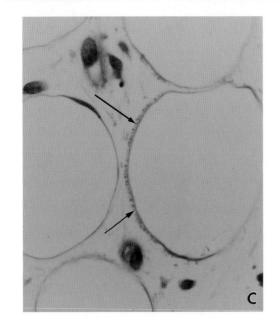
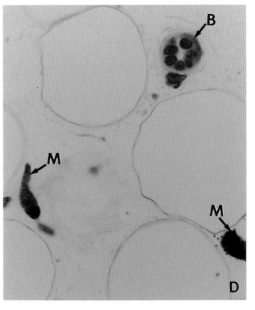

PLATE 179

ADIPOCYTES

A. Mature adipocytes are free of glycogen granules. Glycogen is abundant in the fat of fetal skin and in adipocytes of the hypodermis in the face of young Black women. In some adipocytes, glycogen (arrows) is clustered around the nucleus (N) as well as scattered in the cytoplasm. The presence of glycogen may indicate that these cells are in the process of accumulating fat. From the face of a young Black woman. 4-μm plastic section. PAS lightly counterstained with hematoxylin. OM 400x.

B. This small, immature adipocyte (I) is full of glycogen granules and appears to be accumulating fat. The cell is surrounded by more mature adipocytes (A) in which the glycogen granules are found only in the thin cytoplasm. From the face of a young Black woman. 4-μm plastic section. PAS counterstained with hematoxylin. OM 400x.

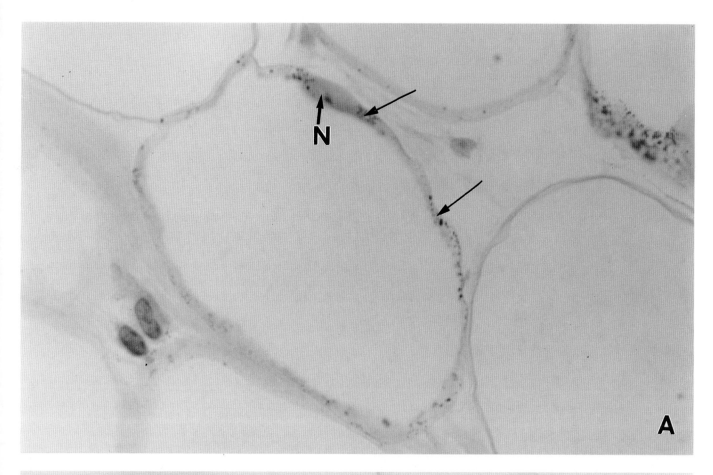

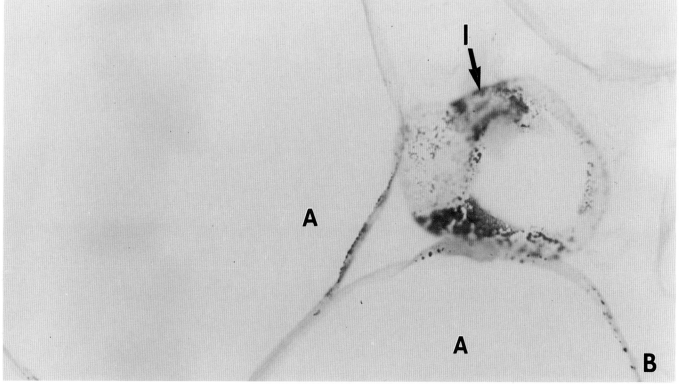

PLATE 180

FATTY TISSUE
Blood Vessels

Fatty tissue around a hair follicle bulb (FB) from the eyebrow of a 12-year-old boy. Only some of the adipocytes are reactive for alkaline phosphatase. During early fetal life, all of the adipocytes are reactive; in adult hypodermal tissue there is little enzyme activity, except in the small blood vessels that supply the tissue. Blood vessels (B). 40-μm frozen section. Gomori's alkaline phosphatase technique. OM 125x.

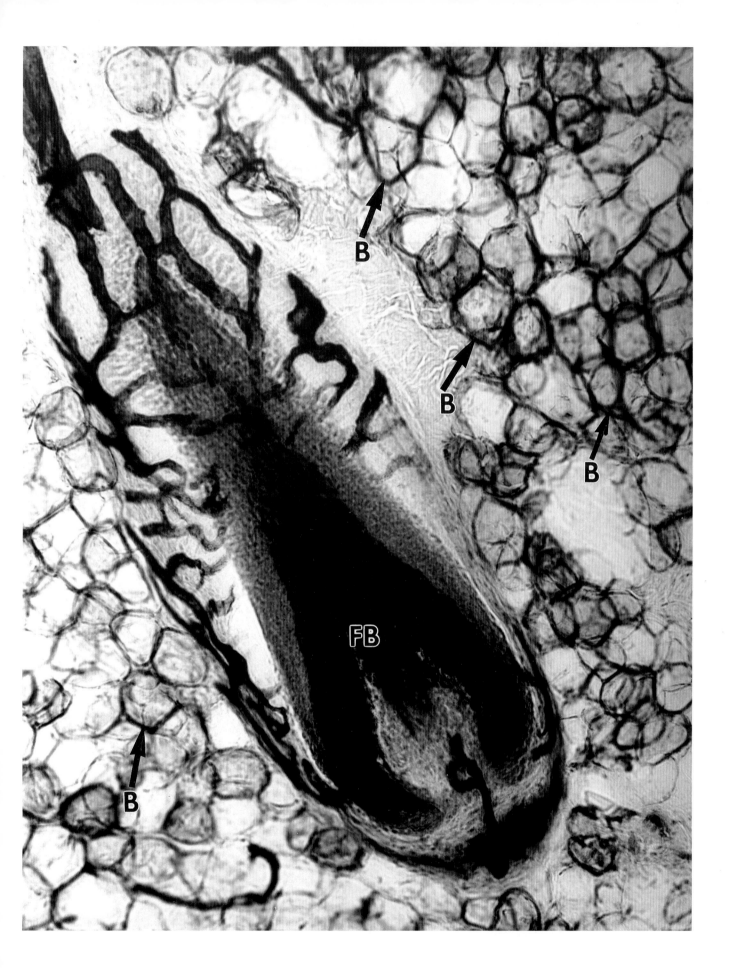

INDEX

Index

Index